Expecting Kindness

Kristin Dibeh has been preparing my clients for childbirth for most of my midwifery career. In my experience her students are knowledgeable and confident. They demonstrate a thorough understanding of the birth process and have the necessary skills to work through an unmedicated labor and birth. In addition, they are prepared to advocate for themselves and for their babies in the rare instance they are transported to the hospital. Kristin has a wealth of information in these pages and if you cannot take her class her workbook is the next best thing.

—Christine Thain, LM

Families that attend Kristin's childbirth education classes are very well prepared for their birth. They feel confident and often report having a great birth experience. I highly recommend Kristin's classes to families preparing for a natural birth.

—Loren Riccio, LM, ND

I have worked with Kristin in many capacities and am continually impressed with the way that she relates to others. Kristin is kind, compassionate and professional at the same time. I highly recommend Kristin as a doula, childbirth educator, and she even teaches my children how to swim in the summer!

—Andrea Henderson, LM, CPM, IBL

I think if I hadn't attended Kristin's wonderful classes my birth experience would have been drastically different. She presents information in a straightforward non-biased way. She answers your questions with kindness. With her help as a teacher and as a doula I was able to have the calm centered natural childbirth I'd hoped for.

She is an amazing teacher, it was money well spent and I would definitely recommend her childbirth classes. The information you'll get will make your birth choices that much easier and less overwhelming. And her skills and generosity of spirit as a doula are invaluable.

—Belinda Philliber

Expecting Kindness

Kristin Dibeh

KIND BIRTH
KIRKLAND WA

ISBN 978-1-939275-05-9

Photo credits:
Jessica Peterson, One Tree Photography, www.onetreephotography.com
Alexis Howe, Life Actually Photography, www.lifeactuallyphotography.com/
Jennifer Reif, photographer
Eastside Birth Center, Bellevue, WA
Autumn & Wes Snow
Elyssa & Matt Cichy
Lucy Nyiri
Melissa & Scott Tuton
Jordan Jensen
Collyn & Isaac Hurst
Shutterstock

Designed by Elder Road Books

*I dedicate this project to my Mom, Darla Eloise Catlin,
who gave birth to me and is the most wonderful mother and friend
in the whole wide world.*

and

*To everyone who has touched my life and inspired me to be my authentic
self; to be the daughter, mother, wife, sister, aunt, friend, mentor,
educator, doula, and the heARTist, that I am.*

Contents

Introduction

I WAS CERTIFIED to teach childbirth education and provide labor support by The American Academy of Husband Coached Childbirth, more commonly known as The Bradley Method, in 1998. I taught this method for about a decade, learning as I went about some of the other great thinkers in the field. I decided to prepare my own workbook based on a broader range of influences and my own experiences teaching and attending births as a labor doula. I've prepared thousands of families for childbirth and attended hundreds of births.

I am an advocate for family-centered, holistic care. Your best chance for an uncomplicated birth is to have a natural childbirth—meaning unmedicated, not just vaginal. This class is designed to prepare couples for natural childbirth. It is clear to me that there is a great misunderstanding regarding why advocates of unmedicated birth, support it so fervently. We are not trying to be superheroes. We are not seeking attention. We are not trying to prove something. We are not seeking self-gratification and bragging rights. We are not deluded, crazy, overconfident, irresponsible, masochistic, hippies. Well, some of us may have been hippies in another ife, but none of these are the unifying factors. We are simply informed, health-focused, strong women who also desire:

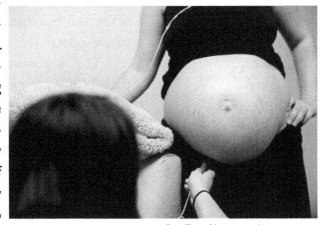

One Tree Photography

1. The healthiest possible baby—a baby who has not been exposed to controlled substances for any reason short of actual medical necessity and who has not been suctioned out or cut out because of frivolous intervention.

2. Control over the experience. The minute you accept an intervention, you relinquish control and accept all interventions that are caused by the first, then the second, and so on.

3. Kindness. We want our care providers to take individualized, holistic care of us, only providing necessary medical interventions. We want the process of giving birth to be honored and respected; we want the family to be the highest priority and the first moments of a baby's life to be calm, warm, and loving.

> We are simply informed, health-focused, strong women.

Intentionally pursuing an unmedicated childbirth by choosing a birth team that supports you, preparing yourself physically, mentally, and emotionally does not guarantee it. Sometimes, for the well-being of mother or baby, a care provider must intervene. Things might not go according to the plan. Your birth plan is a goal. It's like planning for any other important event. Think of it as a physical event, not unlike planning and training for running a marathon. If a runner's feet are bleeding, we don't criticize her for not finishing the race. Conversely, when a runner finishes the race, we don't praise her extraordinary feet because they didn't bleed. That is not a personal failure; it's circumstantial. The whims of nature are evident and acknowledged. Planning a birth is also not unlike planning a wedding. I might trip on my veil as I walk down the aisle, or forget my vows at the altar, but that doesn't mean planning my wedding down to the smallest detail was a failure.

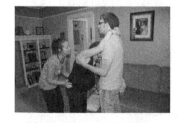

This is a workbook, not a birth education series. It cannot provide the full range of individualized education, entertainment, discussion, or the friendship that can be cultivated in the classroom environment. But the workbook will provide ten weekly lessons that will guide you to an informed birth. Ideally, read and practice these lessons through your third trimester. Each lesson includes a discussion, and online resources including: reading assignments, relaxation exercises, journaling assignments, and exercise suggestions—just like my class.

My philosophy as a birth educator is simple. I want you to have an experience that you can look back on lovingly and without regret, even if your birth doesn't go just as you hope it will. Being an informed consumer and making choices for the health and wellbeing of your child is incredibly gratifying. Sometimes that will mean refusing procedures or treatments that fall into the category of "routine" or "standard procedure" if it is not in the best interest of mom or baby. Sometimes it will mean refusing drugs when they aren't medically indicated even if labor is much harder than you expected. And sometimes for the safety of mom or baby, we have to make decisions to allow interventions, even if you were hoping for an uncomplicated, natural birth experience.

Whatever your wishes, circumstances can be a game changer. Being informed keeps you in the driver's seat. If an alteration to the plan is needed, you are part of the solution, not a victim of it. Your ability to accept deviations from your birth plan will increase if you know for sure they were necessary. Being informed and making decisions using informed consent will allow you to look back at your birth experience and feel like it was your first great moment in parenting.

One last detail: Many activities in the following lessons include a partner or coach. In fact, many segments are written specifically for a partner or other support. It is my belief that this role is essential, but can be provided by a variety of sources. Ideally, of course, your partner is available to you 24/7 and can participate on a daily basis in the planning and preparation leading up to this tremendous physical event. A lot goes on in the hours of labor before most women need to be at their planned birthing facility or until a midwife comes to you. If a partner is inconsistent or unavailable altogether, or you wisely know that a person who has never attended a labor before might need an ally, an informed and supportive mother, aunt, grandma, friend and/or a professional doula can be very effective in filling this role for you. Someone needs to help you with pain management and emotional support during the many hours of labor. If you do not have someone who can be your primary coach, I strongly suggest that you hire a doula.

Doulas are becoming very popular in today's obstetric world. When people ask me about my job, and I say, "I'm a doula," they may

You are not a victim. You are part of the solution.

have heard the term before but most still have no idea what a doula is. Here is what I tell them:

A labor doula is a valuable asset to every birth. The role is incredibly fluid, changing with every woman, every family, and every care provider. There have been times in which I have been the primary support of a single mother, a woman whose partner is out of town on business, out of the picture, uncomfortable with being solely responsible for support, or serving in the military. There have been times when my clients were surrounded by loving support of adoring partners, close friends, sisters, mothers, mothers-in-law, and cousins. There have been intimate births where there was just a midwife and me in attendance. The role changes depending on what the woman and her support team need.

- Some roles the doula plays, include:
- Being a presence with experience.
- Timing contractions, tracking fetal movement.
- Evaluating the progress of labor using external signs and symptoms.
- Facilitating labor progress: using positions/avoiding positions/ encouraging movement/encouraging rest/using visualization/ maintaining hydration and energy/acknowledging and resolving fears by translating the mother's physical sensations and discomforts into the logic of labor progression.
- Creating the desired environment and minimizing discomfort using: conversation or lack thereof, music, candles, deep abdominal breathing, showers or baths when appropriate, aroma therapy, room temperature, keeping the area tidy, keeping certain people present, keeping certain people away, using massage, maternal touch and warm or cold compresses.
- Providing information to help clients to move to their intended birth location or request the midwife to join us at the ideal time.
- Taking pictures or video, or both.
- Assisting the mother in making the transition to the pushing stage of labor, coaching her through until she recognizes the rhythm.
- Physically supporting women in positions when necessary to minimize the strain of holding herself in a squat, for example.

The role of doula changes depending on what the woman and her support team need.

- Informing clients if there are "red flags" indicating a questionable intervention—even if "routine"—or any procedure that departs from the birth plan and helping to ask necessary questions.
- Educating clients about alternatives to routine interventions when possible.
- Educating clients about any undisclosed risks of interventions and the procedures that accompany most routine interventions.
- Advocating for clients who have expressed specific wishes, no matter how few or how many, regarding their care and the care of the new baby.
- Partnering with primary coaches so that they can be in the role that the family wishes for them to be in, in the place where the laboring woman needs them. Knowing in advance what everyone desires from the experience allows the doula to facilitate those wishes and do her best to make your experience as perfect as it can be under any circumstances.
- Having training in emergency childbirth, and the wisdom to avoid using it.
- Helping women/couples understand when a deviation from their desired birth experience is necessary and being informed so that they leave the experience knowing that every question was asked when possible and every alternative was discussed and/or implemented when safe. Her goal is that clients know that no matter the outcome, they made responsible choices for the safety and wellbeing of mom and baby.
- Supporting women immediately postpartum by helping with breastfeeding, continuing advocacy for newborn procedures, and taking care of peripheral responsibilities like ordering food, cleaning up, hydrating mom, photography/videography, bringing in family members, etc. so the family can focus on falling in love.

Of course, an experienced doula is ideal because every birth is continuing education and every mother, a teacher, but do not let the cost hold you back from making sure you are supported. The range of pay begins at $0.00 for a doula who has gone through the certification process, but is lacking experience necessary to be officially certified, and goes up incrementally to nearly $2000.00 depending on geography and years of experience. Want it and can't

"If a doula were a drug, it would be unethical not to use it."
—John H. Kennell, MD

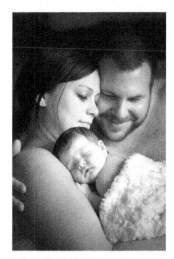

Life Actually Photography

afford it? Make an offer, trade services, make payments, check with your insurance, or use medical reimbursement. It can be kind of expensive, but consider this: if your doula helps you to avoid interventions that increase the risk of Cesarean, she may just have saved you five times her rate, even at the upper end of the pay scale, and supported you in more ways than I can begin to describe. It's hard to really convey the value of having experienced support during the weeks leading up to your labor, the many hours of labor, and birth, and the days and weeks that follow. It is a value that is impossible to recognize until you are in the thick of it, and probably (slightly) over-recognized in the immediate postpartum (I often hear women say that they "couldn't have done it" without their doula) but I have never had a woman say to me that she wished she hadn't had her doula, or that it was an unnecessary expense. Alright, the plug for doulas is over!

Let's begin.

Lesson 1

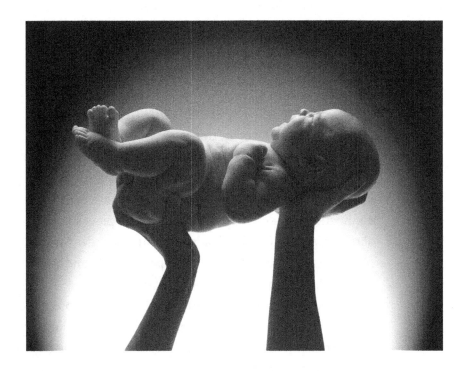

"You are the caretaker of the generations, you are the birth giver," the Sun told the woman. "You will be the carrier of this Universe."

— *Brule Sioux, Sun creation myth*

Overview of Childbirth

Stages of Labor

ONE OF MY favorite things about teaching this class is the nodding of heads as I begin to describe how your body is working throughout the birth process. There is a lot of common sense in uncomplicated childbirth. I love watching future parents make connections when we begin to put all the pieces together and think about how one function leads to another. A new perspective on this process is essential for us to accept it openly and without fear. It is powerful, emotional, and simply beautiful.

Unfortunately, our society teaches us not to trust our bodies, especially surrounding birth. Television shows make birth look like it is either a five-minute, chaotic ordeal or a catastrophic medical condition. It is important to remember that when a comedic character gives birth, it has to take place within a fraction of a show or film, and it has to be funny. Medical shows are the worst, I vividly remember being pregnant with my daughter when ER was running. The solitary episode I watched showed a woman who came to the Emergency Room to deliver her baby. Immediately upon admitting she was diagnosed with: toxemia, pregnancy induced hypertension, gestational diabetes and every other imaginable pregnancy complication. Of course, the Mom doesn't survive and the show closes with the camera panning away from Dad sitting in a rocking chair, holding his motherless child. Cut to me, jaw gaping open, 7 or 8 months pregnant, sobbing. I didn't sleep well for days. This is what we are up against. Media depiction of birth often seems as if the drug lobby is paying for it, commonly normalizing the use of medication and frivolous intervention to the point where I am screaming at the TV like a fanatical sports nut watching my team lose by a million because of a clearly biased ref. These are powerful images and cheap shots that leave a lasting, underlying fear surrounding birth.

One of the core values I want you to take from this series is, "You deserve to be respected, taken care of, treated with nurturing compassion, kindness and, yes, medical expertise." It is reasonable to expect kindness, no matter whether you are with an OB, Family Practice Doctor, or in Midwifery care, and it begins with you. Do not settle for less.

Birth is a normal physiologic process. The woman's body is a miraculous design and <Insert your creation belief system here> did a truly amazing job. The attention to detail is particularly impressive. Labor is, very simply put, the process by which your uterus, a large bag of muscle, contracts in a specific sequence to expel a baby.

Let's begin at the beginning, which can take a variety of forms. It is helpful to have a thorough understanding of "pregnancy anatomy". See "Class Resources" on ExpectingKindness.com for link.

The beginning of labor may be a bit ambiguous, the bag of water can leak, but fluid may also be just cervical discharge, contractions can begin, discomfort in your back from the round ligaments being pulled, Braxton-Hicks like contractions can become more frequent and stronger, loose stool (Mother Nature's way of clearing the pipes), low cramps similar to menstrual cramps. Most of these (barring the obvious large gush of water, however rare) can also be signs of preparation for labor/Pre-Labor/False Labor, or, as I like to call it, a dress rehearsal.

> Trust your body.
> This isn't a television show!

First Stage Labor

FIRST STAGE LABOR is sub-divided into segments based on the intensity and frequency of the muscle contractions: early first stage, active first stage, and transition. In early first stage, labor signs could be subtle and you may not be sure if you are in labor yet. You will begin to see a contraction pattern emerge, if it is to become labor.

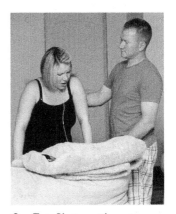

One Tree Photography

Usually, at first, they are spaced far enough apart that it is difficult to make sense of it, there is no need to worry about it until it seems like an obvious pattern. They may be as far apart as 30 minutes or more, or as close as 10, rarely less than 10 at first. You will notice them beginning to last a bit longer and grow a bit stronger, little by little. These warm-up contractions are preparing to pull your cervix open. The cervix is the outlet of the uterus. This early stage of labor always reminds me of trying to turn over a cold engine (being the former owner of a VW Vanagon, you can trust that I know what I'm talking about here). Contractions can start and stop, come in bouts, or turn over and follow a clear ascending pattern becoming progressively closer and stronger. Eventually the engine will rev and you will see significant changes in the frequency, length and strength of your contractions.

As the cervix thins (effaces) opens wider and wider (dilates), the contraction strength has to increase to pull it open further and hold it open. At this stage, you won't be wondering if you are in labor or not; it isn't subtle. This segment of first stage is called active first stage labor, when the cervix changes as we watch. You can imagine a turtleneck sweater, as you put it on. The neck becomes flat against your head (effacement) and then opens to allow the head to move through (dilation). You will begin to notice some discharge tinged with a little blood as capillaries in the cervix are ruptured, this is called "bloody show" and does not hurt. This is the entire function of the first stage of labor: to thin and open your cervix. First stage, on average, takes about 12-18 hours.

Transition is the literal changing, from first stage labor contractions (pulling and holding the cervix open), to the second stage contraction (which is a downward press, expulsive). Here's the kicker… in Transition, you get the pleasure of both for a short time (usually around 15-30 minutes) and although most women report this to be the hardest part of their labor, there is beauty in it, power. As the contractions that are pulling that cervix out of the way are at their strongest, opening it to 8-10 cm and holding it back, the contractions that press down against your baby to move him or her through that opening begin to warm up in just the same way your early first stage contractions did hours earlier. Once the cervix is

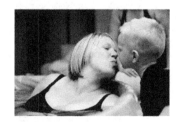

One Tree Photography

completely dilated (also called resolved, complete, gone, 10cm) and once baby passes through the cervix and into the birth canal, those powerful first stage contractions subside. You are left with a new contraction, that downward press, pushing the baby down and out.

This is the end of transition and the beginning of second stage. In my experience, most women (especially women who understand what is happening) really like the change in sensation to pushing.

First stage, on average, takes about 12-18 hours.

Second Stage Labor

SECOND STAGE IS the pushing stage, which is the most commonly misunderstood. We see this stage especially on television with women screaming and shrieking, threatening their partners, flailing about, out of control. The media also has made this stage seem very fast, quite different than what most of my experiences have shown me. The media often confuses strength, power, and effort with pain. Most women are silent/moaning/making some guttural or grunting sounds, and focused during contractions. Then, between contractions, she may be at times: restful, even sleeping, chatting, snacking, and laughing. This stage of labor commonly lasts somewhere between one and four hours.

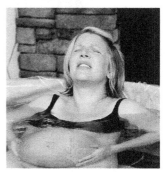

One Tree Photography

Of course, you may have heard about a little thing called crowning, also known as the "ring of fire." I always fight the urge to break into Johnny Cash at about this moment, which I hope is testimonial to my sense of humor and levity in the face if this brief moment of intensity. So, ok, I'm not going to lie to you, it isn't really a particularly enjoyable moment, but it really is just that... it's a moment, sometimes not even that, it is often measured in mere seconds. As the head emerges, centimeter by centimeter, slowly to allow your body to stretch, you will certainly feel a stretching/burning sensation. Your body was made to do this. It is not unnatural.

What you don't often hear about is the joy and excitement inherent in that moment, especially when there is no fear. Women are sometimes able to reach down and touch their baby for the first time, see the hair, know for sure that it is almost over. Looking excitedly into the eyes of their partner and sharing a moment that is indescribable. The physical intensity of the moment is equivalent to the excitement and anticipation of being done and meeting your baby. The tremendous sensation is equivalent to the tremendous relief you feel a moment later. In addition to all of that, you have the added experience of falling in love, instantaneously. It's the incredible swing of physical and emotional intensity that makes this moment unforgettably, incomparably, indescribably beautiful.

And then you fall in love.

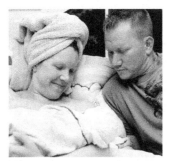

One Tree Photography

Third Stage Labor

AFTER THE BIRTH occurs, we have left second stage and entered the third stage of labor, the expulsion of the placenta. Once the cord stops pulsing (hopefully), your Midwife or OB will clamp the cord in two places, near the baby's belly and an inch or two away to give room to cut in between. After (usually) the cord has been cut, the placenta will detach from the uterine wall on its own (almost always), you will feel some cramps throughout this process and your care provider may need to do some belly/external uterine massage to help the uterus stay firm (contracted), but that is generally the worst of it. The placenta does not hurt when it is expelled; there are no bones in it. You may need to give a couple of little pushes; sometimes little coughs are even enough and then it is pure relief and time to focus on baby!

Homework for Lesson 1

See Classroom Resources on _www.ExpectingKindness.com_ for
Reading assignments
Articles/additional resources
Links to video's
Exercise assignments
Journaling prompts
Tools for partners
Relaxation techniques

Lesson 2

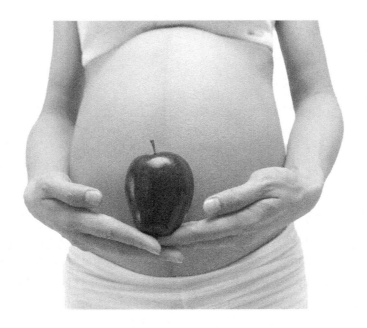

"Nourish Beginnings, let us nourish beginnings.
Not all things are blest, but the seeds of all things are blest.
The blessing is the seed.

Muriel Rukeyser, American Poet

Nutrition and Exercise
to prepare for labor

Nutrition

"LOW RISK." THESE are words that you want associated with you during your pregnancy. We can't control everything, and it is possible for a person in good health, who eats a healthy diet and is physically fit, to still develop pregnancy complications like pregnancy induced hypertension or gestational diabetes. You are responsible for your decisions and avoiding regrets. If a complication arises and you have not practiced good health habits, you will be faced with the following, nagging, unanswerable question: "Could I have prevented this?" However, if you do everything in your power to create a healthy body and something happens anyway, you are free to tell yourself "I did everything I could to prevent this." Then you can accept beneficial treatments or interventions without regret.

Our nutrition discussion assumes you are healthy with a low risk profile. If you have not received prenatal care or are under the care of a practitioner to manage a pregnancy with higher risk, this information may not be directly applicable. Find a qualified care provider and/or discuss any changes with your health professional prior to implementing them. Also, work closely with your care provider to find any resources (nutritionist, naturopath, acupuncture, massage therapy, reiki, reflexology) that may help reduce your risk factors.

Nutrition is a complicated business these days; to eat well sometimes seems like a full-time job. It seems there are as many allergies and sensitivities as there are people, therefore one-size-fits-all programs are impossible. I will provide some resources here and give you some ideas about how you can incorporate simple ideas into your daily routine that will meet your "baby building" needs as well as keep you as healthy and low risk as possible.

The easiest way to be sure you meet your body's needs and your baby's needs is to simplify your diet. Consume whole food or real food only. Don't waste time trying to find "prepared/convenience foods," there is no such thing when it comes to actual health. Eating a healthy diet is easy if you keep it simple. You will, of course, have to make adaptations for vegetarianism, veganism, gluten/dairy/lactose/sugar/etc.-free lifestyles and any other dietary requirements you may have to work with. Balanced diets high in protein grow stronger, healthier babies and keep many pregnancy complications at bay.

Simplify your diet.

You can also use online resources for recipes to increase your protein count while maintaining a well-balanced diet. Dr. Sears has developed an online resource called L.E.A.N. Lifestyle, Exercise, Attitude, and Nutrition, which provides great recipe ideas and information as well as access to workshops and supportive coaches. A diet high in protein but deficient in fats, complex carbohydrates, vitamins or minerals, will not grow a healthier baby, so even if you are only able to eat seventy grams of protein a day (the FDA's recommended daily allowance for pregnancy) within the confines of a well-balanced diet, you will do just fine. When you start tracking your food intake, you will probably find you are consuming more protein than you think you are.

It's important to pay attention to serving sizes when tracking your intake. A serving of animal protein, for example, generally fits inside the palm of your hand. Most Americanized/super-sized servings are far more than three ounces and usually weigh in at least double the recommended serving size, which means at least double the protein content by default. You can also make your daily intake easier by buying "two-fors" or foods that have a serving of both protein and carbohydrate. For example, some breads and pastas have protein and carbohydrates. Some have as many as six grams per serving. Having cereal for breakfast gives you a little protein from the milk, but having oats instead gives you approximately an added ten grams of protein per cup. Add a few cashews or almonds for healthy fat and some milk/almond milk and throw in a few blueberries for vitamin C and antioxidants and you have a very tasty, nearly twenty-gram breakfast in a small, filling meal with vitamins/nutrients, healthy fats, complex carbs and protein. Replacing rice with quinoa is another example, replacing a pure carbohydrate with a grain/protein source.

Keeping it simple and eating real food gets easier with practice and it is an opportunity to model healthy living and eating habits for your growing family. Kids don't always listen, but they see everything you do and will learn by your daily example over the course of a couple of decades!

There is a specific list of foods that have been found to cause harm or have a higher potential of causing harm. I will add this in table format. For specific information, please look up the Center for Disease Control (CDC) and do a search with the keywords "pregnancy and food."

Copy the nutrition tracking worksheet on page 18 as many times as you wish; the more you keep track of your daily intake, the

Foods to Avoid	Because of risks due to
Salt cured/deli/uncooked meats	Listeria bacteria
Unwashed vegetables/fruit	Toxoplasmosis
Fich, uncooked, salt cured	Listeria bacteria
Fish high in mercury	Mercury poisoning
Shellfish, expecially raw	Infection
Raw eggs	Salmonella bacteria
Unpasteurized milks/cheeses	Listeria bacteria
Pate	Listeria bacteria
Caffeine	Calcium deficiency, dehydration, Higher risk of miscarriage, premature birth, low birth weight, and infant withdrawal symptoms
Alcohol	Fetal Alcohol Syndrom and Fetal Alcohol Effects

more intentional you will become. You may also use online resources or smart phone applications if you have a computer or smartphone available, but a piece of paper and a pencil will work just fine.

To help you track your protein intake accurately, the following is a list of foods containing protein and the amount of protein per serving, serving size included. This information has been accumulated from a variety of trusted resources all reporting the same data.

High Protein Foods

Beef

Hamburger patty, 4 oz – 28 grams
Steak, 6oz – 42 grams
Most cuts of beef, 1 oz – 7 grams

Chicken

Chicken Breast, 3.5 oz – 30 grams
Chicken Thigh, average size – 10 grams
Drumstick – 11 grams
Wing – 6 grams
Cooked chicken meat, 4 oz – 35 grams

Fish

Most fish fillets, 3.5 oz – 22 grams

Pork

Pork chop, average – 22 grams
Pork loin or tenderloin, 4 oz. – 29 grams
Ham, 3 oz. – 19 grams
Ground pork, 3 oz. – 22 grams
Bacon, 1 slice – 3 grams
Canadian-style bacon, 1 slice – 5 grams

Eggs/dairy

Egg, large – 6 grams
Milk, 1 cup – 8 grams
Cottage Cheese, ½ cup – 15 grams

Weekly Tracking	Mon	Tue	Wed	Thu	Fri	Sat	Sun
Protein							
Breakfast							
Morning Snack							
Lunch							
Afternoon Snack							
Dinner							
Evening Snack							
Protein Total (70)							
Vegetables/Fruit (3)							
Calcium (4)							
Fish oil (1)							
Eggs (1-2)							
Vitamin C (1)							
Water (63 oz)							

Yogurt (regular), 1 cup – 8-12 grams
Yogurt (Greek style), 6 oz – 15-20 grams
Soft cheeses (mozzarella, brie), 1 oz – 6 grams
Medium cheeses (cheddar, swiss), 1 oz. – 7-8 grams
Hard cheeses (parmesan), 1 oz. – 10 grams

Legumes

Tofu, ½ cup – 20 grams
Soy milk, 1 cup – 6-10 grams
Most beans, cooked (black, pinto, lentil), ½ cup – 7-10 grams
Soy beans, cooked, ½ cup – 14 grams
Split peas, cooked, ½ cup – 8 grams

Nuts/seeds

Peanut butter, 2 Tablespoons – 8 grams
Almonds, ¼ cup – 8 grams
Peanuts, ¼ cup – 9 grams
Cashews, ¼ cup – 5 grams
Pecans, ¼ cup – 2.5 grams
Sunflower seeds, ¼ cup – 6 grams
Pumpkin seeds, ¼ cup – 19 grams
Flax seeds, ¼ cup – 8 grams

Now that you have a good foundation of what to eat and what not to eat, it's time to get to work. Be conscious of what you are putting in your body. Your baby has specific needs in order to grow to his or her full potential. I occasionally have a woman in my class who is concerned about a high protein intake causing a high birth weight. The women that have come through my classroom, participating in this program have rarely shown any fetal growth outside of the range of normal, and genetics are a factor as well. 6.5-9.5 pounds is considered the ideal range of newborn birth weight. "9.5?" you may be gasping. "Yes" is the answer, albeit on the high end of the spectrum, and therefore less common. I get far more worried about the other end of the spectrum because babies born too little are at risk of some challenges in the early days with breastfeeding endurance, complications with jaundice, weight loss, and excessive

Be conscious of what you are putting in your body.

sleepiness. Eat a balanced, high-protein diet, rich in vegetables and fruits, healthy carbs, and fats. You will meet your body's needs as well as your baby's needs, you will limit your risk of diet related pregnancy complications and you will be more prepared for the physical demands of labor. Be well.

Exercise

LET'S MOVE ON to exercise. I will begin with the customary disclaimer. You should always check with your healthcare provider to verify that you are healthy enough to begin any new physical fitness program. Consider it a "sports physical" for your training. Your obstetrician or midwife may suggest variations for particular health concerns, so get the all clear and/or your individualized program prior to beginning. This is by no means an excessive, rigorous prenatal exercise program; in fact, most of the "exercises" are more like glorified positions, but better safe than sorry.

In my experience, these physical assignments are the most commonly disregarded. I can't be there in your living room to create accountability for you, you have to create that for yourself, so along with the description for each exercise, I offer detailed information describing what it does for your body and how exactly it prepares you for childbirth.

The very best advice I can give you is to put your physical fitness at the top of your to-do list and make a commitment to doing a little bit every day. It will quickly become habitual and you won't have to make yourself do it. You have but a few short weeks to train for this challenging physical event. An average labor is twenty-four hours, far longer than your average marathon time; granted you are not working the entire time, you do get breaks, but it is a significant physical challenge nonetheless.

There are some very specific muscle groups that we use more during the labor process than at any other time. If strong, they will be able to carry you through the physical challenges of labor without becoming too fatigued. I will go through these muscle groups one at a time, followed by an exercise to build strength and therefore endurance. Every pregnancy practitioner I have spoken with

Put physical fitness at the top of your to-do list!

Exercise	Mon	Tue	Wed	Thur	Fri	Sat	Sun
Kegel							
Abductor/Adductor fly							
Squat							
Pelvic Tilt							
Cardio							
Stretch							
Relaxation 1							
Relaxation 2							

endorses these exercises; they are universally accepted as beneficial and have been specifically designed with the pregnant woman's needs and safeguards in mind.

Kegel

THE PUBOCOCCYGEUS MUSCLE is known more commonly as the Kegel muscle, named for Dr. Arnold Kegel. It is the muscle that spans the pelvic floor (in both sexes) like a hammock. Its functions include: preventing the prolapse of the bladder (both sexes) and uterus (in women), preventing swelling of the prostate (in men), prevention of urinary and rectal incontinence (both sexes). When it is strong it can increase strength/intensity/duration/control of the sexual orgasm (both sexes).

Do I have your attention? I thought I might.

The Kegel muscle also has a very important job throughout your pregnancy, supporting the growing weight of your baby and then, during labor, your baby moves through the opening in this muscle. The weight of your growing baby requires you to pay special attention to its strength, it needs to be strong to support the baby and (when strong) it helps to avoid the stress on your back, caused by the stretching and pulling of the ligaments that connect the pelvis to the sacrum. Having a toned PC muscle will also prevent having to work much harder to get tone back after labor and birth. It takes a lot more time to build strength than to maintain strength. The baby moving through your pelvis and through an opening in this muscle will stretch it out temporarily and likely cause some mild incontinence following birth, but is certainly recoverable, especially when it is in good tone prior to delivery. To learn to perform a Kegel exercise correctly, you can:

- Try to stop the flow while urinating.
- Insert a finger (yours or your partner's) into your vagina and try to squeeze it.
- Have your partner evaluate your ability to tighten the muscle during sex.

Once you know you have identified the right muscle, you can practice on your own, and explore the benefits together. There is normally a bit of a sex sabbatical following a birth, so enjoy it now!

The hardest part about doing Kegel exercises, is remembering to do them. They are listed on the tracking worksheet on the previous page for you to check off, but rather than waiting till the evening when you are checking off your list, doing them a few times a day is the best way to get them done and build a habit. Try connecting the idea of doing Kegel pulses to something that you do periodically throughout your day. For example, do ten Kegel pulses at every red light or when you are stopped in traffic. At home, do ten Kegel pulses while checking e-mail, talking on the phone, texting, using social media, etc. They are far safer to do while driving than texting or talking is… and it's not illegal to Kegel and drive! Your beginner assignments for Kegel exercise will be listed with the homework each week (online) and will follow an escalating pattern of tensing, holding, an increasing ladder of tension to build strength, but don't limit yourself to these beginner sets, as it becomes easier, try to keep it engaged longer, or do rapid fire pulses, tensing and releasing quickly, or add more reps working your way up to 200, then 400. In addition, you will step down the tension ladder to recognize the sensation of releasing tension and relaxing the muscle to allow the baby to move through the pelvis. It is unfair to your baby to be tightening this muscle as he or she tries to move through it, so learning to relax it is as important as strengthening. It should be toned, and you should be able to consciously relax it.

Hip Adductor/Abductor Fly

THIS EXERCISE BUILDS strength in the adductor and abductor muscles (thigh and hip muscles). Your legs and hips can fatigue as your labor progresses and there is a lot of stress on your hips as your baby descends. Having strong muscles will help support your hips and prevent the shaking that can accompany muscle fatigue.

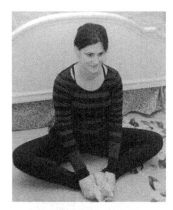

Jennifer Reif, photographer

To do the fly, you sit on the floor; feet planted in front, knees bent. Place your hands, or your partners' hands on the outside of your knees and press your legs open with moderate resistance using arm strength, then place hands on the inside and provide moderate resistance while bring knees back together, or as close together as you can with your baby bump in the way. Variations could include simple Butterfly exercises for hip flexibility and/or side lying leg lifts to build strength. These are large, frequently used muscles and don't take a lot to build strength, so ten of these a day will do.

Pelvic Tilt

THIS EXERCISE WILL engage and build strength in your back, butt, abdominal and core muscles. Having a strong back will support your spine and can minimize discomfort caused by the pulling and stretching on the muscles and ligaments connecting the spine to the pelvis exaggerated by advanced pregnancy as well as labor. Strong abdominal muscles will help support your growing baby, giving your Pubococcygeus (PC/Kegel) muscle some help as well as making it much easier and faster for you to recover your pre-pregnancy core strength. Strong gluteus muscles (maximus and medius) give some stability to the sacrum and coccyx as the baby moves the bones and

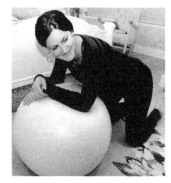

Jennifer Reif, photographer

descends through the pelvis. Additionally, performing this exercise encourages baby into the anterior position, which is the ideal fetal position for birth. Posterior, or "sunny side up" position, causes "back-labor" and makes it harder for the baby to navigate the though the pelvic bones.

To perform the pelvic tilt, position yourself on the floor in the hands and knees position with your hands shoulder width and your knees hip width apart. Head should be neutral. Use your abdominal muscles to pull your baby toward your spine, tilt your pelvis forward, curling toward your belly. Tighten the muscles in your booty and flex the Kegel muscle, hold for five to ten seconds and release. We will be increasing the number of reps you will be performing over the course of a few weeks and then maintaining while you increase your resistance, your growing baby!

Squats

THIS EXERCISE IS meant to increase your flexibility, not necessarily strength training, although there are benefits in both areas. Many women resist the idea of pushing in the squatting position, I'm not sure why. The ironic thing is no matter in which position you choose to push, you will be in a squat. It may be on a bed, with a bar, with footrests, on your side, on a stool, on a ball, in a tub, on hands and knees. Any which way you point your body, your knees need to open wide to give your baby the widest possible opening through the pelvis. Using a full squat position, in addition to all the benefits of opening your knees wide, also gives you the added benefit of gravity as well as the weight of your upper body forcing the pelvis open an additional 10-15%. It also shortens the birth canal, the distance you need to push your baby through. You may not need to use a full squat, perhaps your baby will descend beautifully in a simple reclined position, but even if that's true, flexibility is important. No matter which direction your vagina is facing, your legs will need to be wide open to give your baby as much room as possible. You may be pushing anywhere from one to four hours, every few minutes, it can still be hard on your body if you have been in labor for a while and haven't prepared for holding your body in this position periodically. If you have a baby that takes some effort to move through the

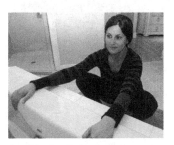

Jennifer Reif, photographer

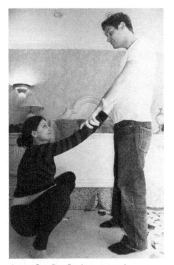

Jennifer Reif, photographer

pelvis and down through the birth canal, the full squat position can become critically important, so not knowing what the pushing stage of labor will require, I like to have people prepare for the most challenging potential outcome.

Having said all that, to do the squat, you simply squat down, legs wide, knees out and try to get your feet flat on the ground. If it's a challenge to get your feet flat, you can lean back against a wall or you can do this with your partner by facing one another, grasping each other's wrists and lowering mama down into a squat, then your partner (standing) can allow you to rock backwards. Slowly work your way to being able to support yourself, flat footed in a full squat. Let your booty sink down as low as possible; like a child picking up pebbles on a beach. The goal is to sink into a squat often throughout the day, letting your inner thigh muscles stretch and get to the point where you can comfortably hang out, bottom relaxed, in that position for 60-90 seconds at a time. Please pay attention and use proper lifting technique getting out of your fabulous squat, if unassisted. Place your hands on your thighs and straighten your knees, then push against your legs to bring your body to upright without straining your back. This is a position that you will find yourself in often with little children, so this can be considered to be part of a physical training for parenting as well. If a full squat is difficult, you may begin using a yoga ball, shift your pelvis forward with feet and legs wide. If your care provider suspects posterior or breech positioning, you may want to avoid a full squat until baby has moved into a head down/anterior position. see resources at www. ExpectingKindness.com and consult with your team for advice/options on helping to encourage better positioning for labor and birth.

Cardiovascular exercise

YOU WILL NEED to choose some form of regular physical exercise that elevates your heart rate but does not exceed the recommended beats per minute (as determined by your care provider) for approximately 20-30 minutes, daily. Feel free to break up the routine with a variety of exercises. I will list my favorites; they are my favorites because they are the most accessible and/or the most transferrable to labor.

- **Walking**. It is easy to work into almost any routine; it can be done outdoors, at home on a treadmill, in a gym, a local school track, or simply walking in place in front of the television.
- **Yoga**. Most people think that yoga is primarily strength training, but trust me, it will elevate your heart rate as well. I love yoga because, like walking, it is something that you can do easily at home, or you can take a class. Additionally, the yogic breath used in yoga is exactly what I recommend using during labor because it oxygenates the bloodstream (and therefore your baby) as effectively as humanly possible and facilitates relaxation. I do recommend that you research your resources and only use a video or an instructor that understands the specific modifications that need to be made for prenatal yoga. It is important to take some natural physical changes in a woman's body into consideration. Consider the lack of a waist when certain bending and twisting positions are required. Consider the (daily) changing center of gravity, making balancing activities riskier. Additionally, yoga will help you learn to have a stronger mind and body connection, listen carefully. What feels good, and why. Could it be useful during labor? As you practice various positions and movements, and learn more about labor, you will begin instinctively and intuitively moving your body in ways that will ease discomforts, while you facilitate the opening of the cervix and the descent of the baby.
- **Swimming**. Swimming is an excellent form of exercise (unless you can't swim) that can be beneficial on many levels. It helps to reduce swelling by re-distributing water (edema) throughout your body, it is great strength training for pretty much all muscle groups, it is unparalleled in cardiovascular training and it feels really, really, really good. You get 30 minutes of feeling not pregnant! Be aware that your center of buoyancy may be different than normal and may take a few minutes to adjust.

There are few types of cardiovascular exercise that I generally advise against, pretty much any sport or activity that involves a good dose of balance or involves a risk of potential/intended impact.

It is not necessary to continuously increase the amount of time you are performing cardiovascular exercise because you are increasing your resistance every day as your baby grows. You will build endurance and have the energy to labor for longer than you would believe. When you are in labor, your body is working like an athlete's; you have endorphins coursing through you. Combining good nutrition, a healthy exercise regimen, and enough fluid intake, your body will have every possible physical advantage to aid you in the pursuit of having an uncomplicated, natural birth.

Homework for Lesson 2

See Classroom Resources on <u>*www.ExpectingKindness.com*</u> *for*

> Reading assignments
> Articles/additional resources
> Links to video's
> Exercise assignments
> Journaling prompts
> Tools for partners
> Relaxation techniques

Lesson 3

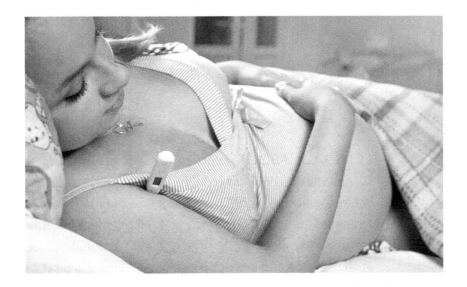

"The most important birthing skill to master is breathing. Breathing is an involuntary, instinctual function that we can learn to control. If you can learn to breathe, you can learn to relax, to open, and to slow your heart rate. If you can learn to control your breath you can learn to control your endorphins. If you can harness the power of your breathing instincts, you can harness the power of your birthing instincts."

Lauralyn Curtis

Contractions and the Art of Breathing and Relaxation

Contractions

LET'S TALK ABOUT contractions. For many women, this word is emotionally charged. The stories we hear from our mothers, grandmothers, co-workers, friends, the media, and even perfect strangers may color the word with so much fear that it can lose its literal meaning entirely. With sustained tension, lactic acid builds up in the muscle and creates a warming, burning sensation and when released, that sensation slowly recedes. You probably don't panic when you push, jump or climb. All of these activities involve muscle contractions.

The sensation of a uterine contraction is no different than any other muscle group; the uterus is a large muscle, a bag of muscles close to the size of a small watermelon. The sensation of uterine contraction is similar to the abdominal muscles, so imagine doing an isometric abdominal crunch, or holding yourself in plank pose for a minute or two. You can feel the muscle begin to tighten, as you hold the position, a warming sensation begins to spread across your abdomen. As time passes that warming intensifies into a burning sensation, you are tempted to release it, but want a good workout so you continue to tense the muscle. Your breath increases, deep breaths in through the nose and out through the mouth to get through the intensity. Finally, you reach your target of 60 seconds and you release the tension. The burning slowly descends back down to that familiar warmth and as you relax between sets the sensation dissolves entirely.

Welcome to labor contractions. The uterine muscle is a strong three-dimensional Pyriform (pear shaped) muscle, not a flat, two-dimensional muscle, and is therefore more powerful, which naturally produces stronger sensations. As labor progresses, your contraction will become stronger than any muscle contraction you have felt before. I avoid the use of the word pain as much as possible. The tremendous sensations you feel during a normal labor progression are different than the pain of kidney stones, menstrual cramps, broken bones, sprains, migraines, tendonitis, torn meniscus, back or neck pain/injury etc. While it might hurt at times, the experience is different in four very important ways.

1. You get rests.
2. It is predictable.
3. It is imminently purposeful.
4. You get a baby.

Rests: In the beginning the rests far outweigh the actual time laboring, sometimes 20 minutes rest to 30-45 seconds contraction. That ratio will shift over hours and by the time you are in active first stage through transition, the rest to contraction ratio is one of the bigger challenges. In addition to the physical challenge, there is an added emotional element; not knowing how long you will be doing this hard work may increase your perception of difficulty. It's like running a race in which you do not know the terrain of the course, and you do not know exactly where the finish line is, but the rests between contractions are an undeniable respite.

Predictable: In the beginning of first stage labor, you may not even have to interrupt a conversation to have a contraction; they begin like little waves and usually increase gradually, over many hours with periods of climbing intensity and periods of plateau. The peaks of the waves come on stronger and last longer, but will sustain the wave-like sensation until Second stage, when the sensation changes completely and the rest to contraction ratio flips, longer rest periods/shorter contractions. The contraction progression of

You get rests.
It is predictable.
It is imminently purposeful.
You get a baby.

first stage is similar to gradually increasing the incline while walking on a treadmill. When you press that button and the incline increases, maybe 20%, it is noticeably different but after a few minutes, you adapt your breathing, you reach a plateau and can keep going. You may stay there for a while and then realize you can increase it again, another 20%, seems challenging at first, but you adapt again, and again, and again. Labor is really like a bad-ass personal trainer. Pushing you farther than you thought you could go; farther than you would ever push yourself.

Purposeful: Labor contractions bring pain, but not pain that is telling you that something is wrong. It is telling you where your baby is. It is massaging and preparing your baby for life outside the womb. It is telling you what to do to facilitate the birth. Your baby and your body are communicating with each other in the only way they can, physically and intuitively. We can choose to think of them as negative or fearful things happening to us

> *OR*

Positive, powerful, creative forces that are a part of us.

I choose B.

Baby: Babies are awesome. The depth of love you will have for this life is unlike any other love. It is unimaginable. It is so powerful that your own life will seem infinitely more valuable, because it has a tremendous purpose. It feels like a whole new chamber of your heart just burst spontaneously into existence and beats for your baby alone. It takes nothing away, but adds depth to every experience. It's as if everything becomes re-enchanted, like you are experiencing life for the first time, through their eyes. In short, he or she is worth it, a million-fold.

Most kinds of pain don't offer a reward at all. The most you may get is a great story, a scar, maybe a little pebble in a jar. In the huge swing from intensity, to a beautiful release, to instantly falling in love, there is a huge range of unparalleled physical experience and human emotion. It is unlike anything else you will ever experience. Even in the case of an unwanted Cesarean section, which is simply a different kind of birth, there is a unique range of beauty and emotion. The birth of your baby will create a memory that you will treasure, even if it doesn't look exactly the way you anticipated.

Having the conviction to experience your labor is a very important part of actually having a natural childbirth. There are no guarantees of course, but this isn't exactly something you can just try to do. If you value the experience, or seek an uncomplicated experience for health or personal reasons, you must prepare. You wouldn't just try to run a marathon or compete in a triathlon; you must train for it. You plan for the anticipated discomforts and have the tools and support available to you during the event. I have two simple tools for you aside from the physical preparation we have already covered. They are breathing and relaxation.

Breathing

YOU HAVE PRESUMABLY been breathing naturally as you have been reading this section, so let's take a moment and observe your natural breathing and compare it to intentional breathing. Breathe naturally for ten cycles of inhalation and exhalation, pay attention to what part of your body rises and falls, do you have a natural pause? If so, where is it? Is it the peak of inhalation or the depth of exhalation? Keep that in mind as you read on and then we will go through a guided yogic breathing sequence so you can really observe the difference.

Visualize the oxygen as you inhale, entering your lungs, saturating your blood, which then carries that oxygen to every part of your body.

Often, we are not great breathers in our current culture of business, activities, hard play, multi-tasking, and not enough rest. We often awaken in a panic, rush through our over-scheduled daily routines, and even try to hurry to sleep at night. Even if we didn't change our existing pattern, but added in intentional, deep breathing exercises periodically throughout our day, we would function better. Every cell in your body (as well as your baby's body) requires oxygen to perform its job.

You, as a whole, perform no better than the smallest particles of your body. You can survive on hurried, shallow breaths, but optimum performance requires deep circulation of oxygen in your system.

Visualize the oxygen as you inhale, I like to imagine tiny particles of light, entering your lungs, saturating your blood, which then carries that oxygen to every part of your body. As your blood passes by the placenta, the oxygen (and everything else you put into your system) passes into your baby's bloodstream. As we go through the yogic breath sequence, you will likely feel your baby move or kick. Baby is telling you that he or she likes the added O2. Breathing is a very important skill to master.

To sum up all the benefits: Deep breathing is more conducive to relaxation. The shallow breath/panic/pain cycle is interrupted when you slow your breathing. You are better able to release added, discomfort-causing tension. Your body will perform all the necessary functions of labor better if it is well oxygenated. In labor, we can literally watch the baby's heartbeat accelerate with deep breathing and decelerate with shallow breathing. If you need another reason to practice deep breathing, it is a skill you will absolutely need throughout your parenting career. My children are adults and I still use it daily, several times a day, usually to interrupt the terrible and useless habit of worry.

Master this skill: The Yogic Breath
TO BEGIN, OBSERVE your natural breathing for ten cycles.

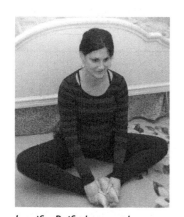

Jennifer Reif, photographer

Abdominal breathing
As you continue to breathe naturally, notice how your abdomen rises slightly with each inhalation and then falls as you exhale. Focus on your abdomen and begin to intentionally breathe deeper, gently bulging your abdomen outward as you inhale, and feeling it collapse inward as you exhale. Continue to practice for two minutes, approximately twenty breaths.

Thoracic (chest) breathing
Return to your natural breathing pattern, but now turn your attention on to rise and fall of your chest. Take five breaths with this focused observation.

Now begin to extend your inhalation, try to increase the rise and expand your rib cage. As you exhale, try to empty the lungs completely. Continue this practice for two minutes, approximately twenty breaths.

Yogic breathing

We will now combine the above two steps. You will begin with your abdominal breathing and then, imagining a motion similar to a wave, continue to inhale as you extend the breath into your chest. Allow for a pause at the peak of inhalation if it feels natural to you. Then reverse the wave, exhaling first from the chest, allowing your lungs to empty and then wringing the air all the way down through the abdomen. Allow for a pause at the depth of exhalation if it feels natural to you. Repeat the whole cycle for two minutes, approximately twenty breaths. You may feel a little euphoric, it's almost as if breathing deeply is important and healthy, and were rewarded with a good feeling.

It will take practice to master this skill, try to spend time breathing intentionally several times a day, and use it to combat stress, wind down before bed, during your relaxation practice, and to connect with your baby. Daily practice will make it easier to apply this skill during labor contractions, which is important for many reasons. First, relaxation decreases pain. Second, your body is working hard and needs to be well oxygenated. Third, during uterine contractions the flow of oxygen through the placenta is decreased, causing a normal deceleration in your baby's heart rate. Using yogic breathing during, as well as in between, contractions will give your baby the highest possible level of oxygenation in his or her bloodstream, thereby decreasing the risk of fetal distress. And finally, you will use this skill for years to come, perhaps in future births and certainly in the middle of the night trying to nurse your newborn, trying to teach your growing baby new skills, putting your child on the school bus for the first time or teaching them at home, seeking patience for positive parenting/discipline, watching them learn to swim, play football, drive a car, graduate, go to college… A lifetime of slow, deep breaths awaits you.

Try to spend time breathing intentionally several times a day.

Relaxation and Massage

SOUNDS SIMPLE. MOST people believe that they can relax because they fall asleep at night. While this is true on a very superficial level, it takes more than that to be able to respond to labor

There are three different types of relaxation to consider: sensual, mental, and emotional.

contractions with relaxation. Let's relate labor once again to an athletic event. This time we'll use cycling. In this scenario, the muscles of the legs will play the part of the uterus. Most people can get on a bike and ride for a while, perhaps even climb a hill or two. True cyclists, those who ride to work every day or compete in races have used knowledge and practice to

1. Build strong muscles used to pedal and support the body.
2. Build cardiovascular endurance.
3. Use only the amount of energy that is absolutely necessary by intentionally relaxing all other muscles in the body.

This allows the blood flow to be drawn to the muscles required to perform the actions needed. If you have ever watched the Tour de France, you may have noticed that those guys don't even use energy to spit or to "hold it" if you know what I mean. Saliva just trails out of their mouths and the pee flows freely. Gross? Kinda. Effective? Absolutely. Imagine the focus that is required to relax all the muscles in your body that are not specifically required to climb the French Alps, while climbing the French Alps. Maybe more relatable analogy is relaxing your whole upper body, while doing a wall-sit for 60 seconds, go ahead and try it. Legs at a 90-degree angle. Now, relax your face, the muscles around your eyes, your neck, your jaw, your shoulders, the muscles in your back, let your arms hang loosely at your sides. Falling asleep at night is probably sounding simple now. Intentional relaxation during a physical event takes some real internal evaluation and then a real investment of time and attention. It may seem like a big commitment, but these are skills that you will carry with you into positive parenting and any other physical challenges you *will* face in your life.

There are three different types of relaxation to consider: sensual, mental, and emotional.

Sensual relaxation

SENSUAL RELAXATION INVOLVES engaging the senses in ways that are calming, allowing you to reach a state of total physical relaxation. Massage is often at the top of this list. There are some specific massage techniques that will be included in the weekly relaxation assignments, but I want to talk a little about labor massage because it can be intimidating for birth partners if they don't feel like they are particularly gifted in this area. I often see a few partners rolling their eyes when I use the word massage—it seems like they might be thinking that you've roped them into this class just to get a daily massage, mandated by yours truly.

Partners, you absolutely do not need to be a licensed massage practitioner to perform massage during labor. Labor massage is usually very simple and repetitive, with a few slight variations as labor progresses. Sometimes, your hands on her body so she knows you are there is all the touch that is necessary—sometimes more. Practice each day is recommended and here's why. As a primary support person, you will be there during the early hours of labor, before a doula (if you have one) and certainly before your Midwife or Doctor. She will need some trained support; it's not the time to be guessing at where she might hold tension or at how she likes to be touched. There is a certain amount of learning through practical application that can be taken care of ahead of time so that when she needs you—and she will—you are ready. Think of her as your athlete; as her coach, you wouldn't expect any other athlete to show up on game day and perform well without having worked with their coach in advance.

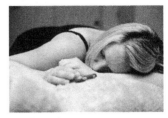

One Tree Photography

The type of massage we'll use the most is simply a guiding technique. The pressure is an important factor; not so light that it tickles and not so hard that it is a distraction. With Mom lying on her side, begin at the neck or shoulders and, using moderate pressure, move the tension down her arms and out of her body. The stroke should end at the tips of her fingers so she can clearly feel the tension leaving her body. You can use the same technique on her legs, beginning at the hip and stroking down to the tip of her toes. You can usually get several full strokes in within a contraction. There will be more examples in the chapters discussing the specific stages of labor with tips on when to apply different techniques. In order to realize all the benefits, practice is essential.

Another sensual tool is verbally guided relaxation. This one is sometimes hard to practice because people "feel silly." So, what? Feel silly, allow it to be funny, but practice the techniques in the homework assignments because some women really need verbal

Feel silly, allow it to be funny, but practice the techniques.

guidance to maintain their breathing, to relax each muscle group by drawing her attention to it, to not feel alone, and to get through tough contractions. Other sensual relaxation tools you have available are: Room temperature, body temperature (using blankets, hot water bottles, showers, baths, cool compresses), candle light, nourishment with food and water (I once spoon fed a woman chocolate during her transition—tiny little bites melting in her mouth between contractions. I thought that was brilliant!), fragrances that feel calming, and relieving unnecessary pressure by emptying your bladder frequently. You can create an environment that is, for lack of a better word, romantic. A soft, loving, comforting, sensual environment creates a sense of security that will help her allow the labor to take over.

Mental relaxation

MENTAL RELAXATION GIVES you specific things to concentrate on during, or in between, your contractions. For many women, music is a very important element. Making a "labor playlist" is a fun project to do as a team, but the laboring party gets two votes.

Visualization is another mental relaxation tool that sometimes seems silly during practice because the language may be unfamiliar. It might seem funny to talk about consciously relaxing your pelvis. But you can do it. Women who tense the Kegel muscle and the muscles around the vagina, called the perineum, during contractions are working against the objective. It makes the job the uterus is trying to perform harder than it needs to be. By using visualizations that allow her to see progress—softening the Kegel and relaxing the perineum—she is facilitates the birth process instead of challenging it. These visualizations can be concrete like, "Imagine your cervix opening, softening," or more abstract like, "Picture a tight flower bud, opening toward the sun." These are personal preferences, women will gravitate to some and not others. That's why it's important to do some practice. If you are not a "flower imagery" kind of girl, you will want your support team to know that prior to labor. Active labor (when these tools are applied) isn't the time to be experimenting, it will be distracting and make contractions harder for her, and it is truly no fun to get to the most challenging

It is the job of your support team to make sure that you have an environment that isn't distracting.

part of her labor, only to realize that you don't know how to ease her discomfort. Load your toolbelt.

Emotional relaxation

EMOTIONAL RELAXATION CERTAINLY has to do with how you feel about what is going on inside your body, reminding women, especially as labor progresses into late first stage and transition. Reminding her what the sensations mean, giving her a map, assuring her that she is making progress and making sure she knows that she is not alone are all critical.

Very often, though, emotional relaxation has more to do with what is going on around you. One element of emotional relaxation involves avoiding distractions. Active labor contractions take a good deal of focus; it is the job of your support team to make sure that you have an environment that isn't distracting. Some common distractions include: People entering and exiting a room frequently and/or noisily, casual conversation, incessant questions, phone's ringing/text notifications, undesirable music, touch that is: too soft, too hard, too unpredictable, machines beeping, cords, straps, and pelvic examinations.

Checking the cervix. This is a practice that really requires us to be in control of our own bodies. I usually suggest an "exit only" policy, and then your providers are required to authentically ask you permission before checking your cervix. The habit of checking on your dilation is outdated and largely unnecessary. When a woman can be 1 centimeter dilated and give birth in a few hours, OR she can be one centimeter dilated and give birth in a week, tell me, what does 1cm mean? If a woman can be 6cm dilated and give birth in an hour, or she can be 6cm dilated and give birth in 18 hours, what does 6cm mean? If your provider is a fan of checking your cervix, especially prenatally, I'd strongly advise that you have "the talk". The "exit only" talk. They will still advise you if there is an actual medical reason to check you, but most of these exams are performed for no valid reason, and there are risks. A spike in adrenaline caused by anything, really, can slow the labor process and even stop it. Fear, anxiety, pain from exams, and even excitement (good or bad) are virtual enemies of the progress of labor. You may be thinking "I wonder if this is related to the high Cesarean section rate?" If so, the answer is yes. There is no question in my mind that it is a factor in the equation.

You must control the birth environment in order to be emotionally relaxed, which brings us back to maintaining the "low risk profile" as much as humanly possible. Once an intervention has occurred, it becomes more difficult to be in control. The intervention itself elevates your risk level; you have given someone else the right to manage your labor. Your desires and childbirth plan become a much smaller factor in the equation. They may still be considered, but will be at the discretion of the practitioner. Now, this particular subject has a way of bringing up an important topic: choosing your birth team and location.

Choosing your birth team and location

A KEY FACTOR in being able to manage the emotional and physical stress of labor is having the right environment for your baby's birth. Even if you believe that you have your team in place, please read this so you are well-informed as you discuss your birth plan with them.

Choosing your birth environment is a critically important decision for you to make. The environment that you choose and the care provider you have with you during labor have the power to make or break your ability to achieve the level of calm and relaxation you need to be able to handle the escalating challenge of labor contractions. I will be speaking in broad terms, sharing my personal experiences here. It is opinion based on experience. You may use this information as you wish.

There are only a few options available to you in regard to your birth team. An OB, an in-hospital midwifery team (CNM or Certified Nurse Midwife), an independent Licensed Midwife, an M.D. or Family Doctor, and in some cases a Perinatologist. (If you are in a higher risk category, you may wish to include a Perinatologist on your team. They specialize in high risk. Therefore, any minor risk factors will be perceived as largely, well, boring by comparison to what they are accustomed to. That can be a real advantage.)

You may feel comfortable with your OB/Gyn and have a long history with him or her in your gynecological care, but these two roles are very independent of one another and therefore you cannot assume that his or her philosophy of labor and birth is aligned with yours. I often hear women say they are seeing a practitioner because of a recommendation from a close friend, that's fine as long as your friend shares your ideals for childbirth and had a supportive experience with that person.

Some women hesitate to interview a Midwife because they think it is too far out on the fringes—too "woo-woo." Midwives today are medical professionals. They don't all flit about in peasant clothes and swing incense around the room, although they might if it was important to you! In any case, you can't make any kind of an informed decision by relying on non-relevant experiences (loyalty to your gynecologist), the non-relevant experiences of friends or family (blindly hiring your friends OB), or outdated stereotypes (as with a hippie midwife). It is critically important to interview different care providers with the mindset of hiring an employee. Come armed with a list of interview questions for all potential care providers. Additionally, I would encourage you to not make a final decision in the moment, even if you really like one of them. That person will still be there tomorrow. A good practitioner in any of these fields will appreciate you taking responsibility for your own wellbeing. An undesirable provider may be defensive, controlling, and threatened. Knowing that you have extensively interviewed and made an informed choice about your care provider can be incredibly reassuring, which in turn should give you a sense of peace, helping you achieve relaxation in labor.

Hold on to your original interview questions and answers, to refer to them later if you feel that your practitioner has changed his or her tune. Some practitioners will simply tell you what they think you want to hear. Feeling unsure of your environment and having reservations about the people caring for you does not facilitate your labor progression. It is also very important to know that if you decide to change care, you don't have to "break up" with your OB/Gyn. If you change care to another OB, or to a different midwifery practice, their office will generally just send a records request to

> Take responsibility for your own wellbeing. Ask questions!

your previous providers office staff, they fax it over and you simply don't make another appointment. You can also kindly and plainly leave a message, if you wish, stating that your wishes for your birth are aligned better with a different practitioner but that you would like to continue your gynecological care. It's business, not personal. Even though we tend to feel personal about those who are involved with this intimate kind of care, for them, it is mostly a job. If they really care, they will want you to be where you feel the safest, even if it isn't under their care.

Hospital

Benefits

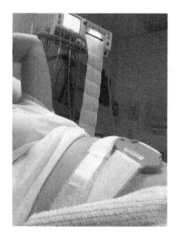

There are amazing, considerate, and kind obstetricians out there; I have had beautiful birth experiences with many OB's who clearly get the value of good care, patience, trust, support and security in a healthy labor. There are obvious benefits to being in a hospital environment if you have a complicated pregnancy that may prevent a birth free of intervention: Access to monitors, medications, perinatal and neonatal staff, and the operating room. There are also some women who don't feel safe in an out-of-hospital environment and that is a valid reason for pursuing conservative care in a supportive hospital environment so long as the decision isn't being made out of misinformation or presumptions or baseless fears. I am not in the business of demonizing the hospital, staff, or surgery. They are brilliant, magical, beautiful, and heroic…when we choose carefully and when they are necessary.

Risks

If you are planning a hospital birth on a "just in case something might go wrong" basis there are some particular risks. The hospital is a business, a finely tuned machine that has a very ingrained standard of care. If it doesn't align with your intentions for your birth, you are likely fighting an uphill battle. It is possible to win the battle against policy driven care as long as you are informed and there are no complications, but it doesn't have to feel like a battle. There are other hospitals, other doctors who will offer you what you are looking for. If you are serious about having an empowered, intervention free (as much as possible) birth, you have to become your own medical advocate. Make sure that you have the provider you think you do by asking challenging questions. A good OB will like the challenge and will not be offended. In contrast, if he or she (or a partner) becomes defensive, controlling, or angry with your inquisition, thank them for their time and don't make another appointment. Find someone else. The best chance for an uncomplicated birth in a hospital environment is through choosing your birth team extremely carefully.

You are not sick! You're pregnant.

Some OB's are simply surgeons, they just like to do what they were trained to do. They don't feel it is a disservice to their client. A Cesarean Section is considered by some OB's to be an option in childbirth, not the last resort. It is more convenient to schedule, less time consuming (a Cesarean takes only about 30 minutes from start to finish), gives them a much larger paycheck than a long, unmedicated vaginal birth, and it allows them to use the skills and tools that they have tirelessly trained to perform. It gives them something to do other than wait. Under any other circumstance, it's the way we want our surgeons thinking. They view body processes as a series of functions: compression, valves, tubes, and shafts, like plumbing. It shouldn't be terribly difficult to identify this breed of care. These practitioners show their colors pretty openly during an interview, they often take pride in it. You are likely to hear phrases like; "I'm willing to let you try," "I'm willing to allow," "I don't like birth plans, I prefer birth preferences," "I'm concerned that you will be disappointed if you have such high expectations." They also are known for laying the foundation for the need to intervene throughout your prenatal course. They will raise concerns prior to any kind of actual (or even remote) diagnosis, creating an underlying sense of fear without cause, regarding: the size of the baby, the size of your pelvis, the amount of fluid, baby's position, etc. People who are afraid are easy to manipulate. If you experience this, again, thank them for their time and don't make another appointment, find someone else.

There is another root cause of unnecessary intervention that we need to acknowledge and take responsibility for. Our litigious society has created a dangerous trend in obstetrics. If a surgeon performs every intervention possible, and something still goes wrong, that surgeon can prove that he or she did everything in their power and their ability (however unnecessary) to prevent a negative outcome. Ultimately, that means they can defend themselves in the event that malpractice is alleged against them. The risk of losing a malpractice suit is higher for the Doctor if he or she doesn't react to any and all signs (even if they could be normal) that could potentially be linked to any complication. This isn't a good reason to throw every intervention at every labor. Every intervention carries its own potential risks that wouldn't otherwise exist, but a doctor is not penalized for doing more than necessary even if it causes harm or creates risk.

When you sign on the dotted line upon admission, you essentially waive their responsibility for over-treating. As a society, we need to reevaluate our need to assign blame in the event that there is an undesirable outcome—even when there is a human error. Malpractice is a term that actually means "negligent conduct" for the mother or baby in the case of obstetric care. Exactly how often do OB's knowingly and intentionally put a mother or child in danger? Really. My guess is the statistic of actual disregard is significantly lower than the rate of suit. Of course, it happens, that is why we have malpractice insurance, but negligence is a strong word, and lawsuits are making it ever harder for OB's to practice without fear, and fear causes excessive use of practices that are not appropriate for a healthy labor. The reality is that no one gets any kind of guarantee with regard to the health and wellbeing of their baby. Ever. It's scary, but the truth is I have no more of a guarantee today with my adult children, than I had the day they were born. Frivolous lawsuits are destroying the health care system on which we rely.

The following is a list of questions to ask your obstetrician. In some cases, we really want the answer, in some cases we just want to see how they react. You should trust your intuition above all.

Questions to ask your OB/Gyn and in-hospital Midwifery practice:

Begin with a statement of your intent. Something like:

"I have a number of questions and would appreciate very clear, specific answers. I am seeking an OB who is willing to work with

Keep these questions and answers to refer to if you feel your practitioner has changed his or her tune.

Questions to ask your OB/Gyn and in-hospital Midwifery practice:

1. What is your experience attending unmedicated labor?
2. Do you offer a water birth option? If no, why?
3. What is your opinion about having a birth doula?
4. What (specific or estimated) percent of your patients deliver without any of the following interventions?
   - Induction with Pitocin
   - Epidural/Spinal Anesthesia
   - Morphine
   - Continuous Fetal Monitoring
   - Cesarean Section
     What percentage of c-sections would you consider to be low risk pregnancies?
   - Limited pelvic exams
   - Forcep or vacuum extraction
5. What classes do you recommend for people seeking an informed birth?
6. Can I request a nurse that has experience supporting unmedicated labor?
7. Do I have the right to refuse nonessential staff being present at visits and/or delivery?
8. What would you consider to be routine procedure under your care?
9. In the event of a non-emergency situation that requires us to consider a deviation from our birth plan, I would like to give informed consent. Are you comfortable answering questions so I can be a part of the decision-making process?
10. I realize the option for pain management exists and I may ask for it if necessary. If requested, will you commit to not *offering* medication? Will you challenge me by offering alternatives? Will you help me understand if the intensity is due to approaching transition or significant progress, discouraging medication if it isn't medically necessary?
11. What are your policies or opinions about alternative pain management techniques like:
    - Sterile water injections: An intracutaneous injection of sterile water near the sacrum which alleviates back pain in labor for up to two hours and can be repeated as necessary.
    - TENS: A pad placed in 4 location around the sacrum which deliver an electric pulse which increases the production of serotonin and activates the opioid receptors creating a mild analgesic effect without using controlled substances.
    - Acupuncture (if provided)
    - Massage
    - Freedom of movement

- Eating/drinking lightly to maintain endurance
- Bath/Shower
- Nitrous Oxide: Not used widely in the US, yet, but popular in many other developed countries.

I want you to begin to normalize the conversation about the use of Nitrous Oxide for women in labor because it is far safer than Opiate and Caine derivative drugs currently used to manage normal labor discomforts in the U.S. Let's save the controlled substances for surgery and last resort pain management.

12. What is your experience working with patients who have a detailed birth plan with clear objectives, goals, and desires?
13. How many births have you attended?
14. How many labors (from first stage to birth) have you witnessed and/or attended?

me and help me make informed decisions. I understand that complications sometimes arise, and I am not intending to challenge your medical expertise in the event of an emergency. We will, of course, be willing to deviate from any plan in the event that it becomes truly healthier to intervene. My questions are pertaining to an uncomplicated labor."

Some practitioners may try to deflect your questions by bringing up hypothetical emergencies. Steer them back to normal birth and wait patiently for specific answers, repeating the question if necessary. If they resist answering a question or act as if it isn't relevant or claim they don't know their own statistics, there is probably a good reason. Listen to what they don't or won't say as much as to what they do say.

Out-of-Hospital Birth

Benefits

Licensed Midwives (LM) are becoming very common, though not every community has a free-standing birth center. You are likely to find at least a handful of Midwives who either have privileges at a local hospital or offer home birth care. In the face of a normal, uncomplicated pregnancy and labor, the prenatal care of an experienced, caring LM or Certified Nurse Midwife (CNM) is more personal than OB care. The visits are generally longer, giving you enough time to really get to know one another, develop trust, feel you have been heard, ask all your questions, express your fears and resolve them, create a circle of support, and meet all potential attendants so there are no strangers in the room. Midwives generally have more experience with fostering a calm environment so you feel secure and can let labor take over.

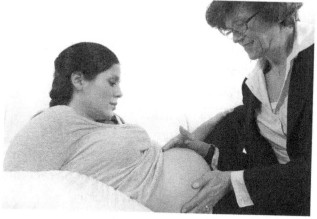

The atmosphere at home or in a freestanding birth center is non-threatening. Generally, they do not even offer most of the "services" we wish to avoid. Midwives are likely to have more experience with normal labor than an OB will. They are trained for and have attended hundreds or thousands of low-risk, uncomplicated births. It is truly an entirely different profession.

Risks

There is a possibility you will need to be transported to a hospital or have your care escalated to an OB. Most complications that would warn against midwifery care are evident during your prenatal care or are non-emergency during labor. You will still have access to your midwifery team's relationships with or knowledge of local practitioners in the hospital. Most transports to the hospital

---

Questions to ask your out-of-hospital Midwife

1. How long have you been practicing?
2. How many births have you attended?
3. How many Midwives are there in your practice?
4. Will I have the opportunity to meet with all potential birth attendants including any students or assistants?
5. How long have they been in practice?
6. Can I request to not have students actively giving care?
7. Where did you receive your education?
8. Are you a Licensed Midwife? A CNM?

9. What percentage of your care is covered by my insurance and do you offer a payment plan for the balance?
10. What do you consider to be your strengths?
11. What can you tell me about your personal philosophy regarding my care before and during my labor?
12. How long is a prenatal visit?
13. What is your opinion of a birth plan?
14. What would fall into the category of routine procedure under your care?
15. What kinds of pain management do you offer?
    - TENS
    - Sterile water injections
    - Nitrous Oxide
16. Do you have a Doula on staff or recommendations?
17. What is you rate of transport?
18. Tell me about what a non-emergency transport looks like.
19. Tell me what an emergency transport looks like.
20. What are the most common reasons for transporting?
21. Do you have a back-up OB or relationships with supportive obstetricians in case of a transport?
22. Do you accompany me to the hospital if a transport occurs?
23. Do you have recommendations for a childbirth education class?

during labor are non-emergency, meaning that a factor has come up that requires additional care, but doesn't necessarily require immediate emergency medicine or surgery. Occasionally emergency transport is necessary for the health and wellbeing of Mom or baby and in that case the closest hospital offering Obstetric care is the obvious choice. There may not be time to ask a million questions or make accommodations for the aromatherapy you wanted, but under these circumstances the priorities are reevaluated and we simply do what needs to be done. Every intervention, up to and including Cesarean, has benefits when they are medically indicated.

The midwifery movement is growing and becoming mainstream, but practices are still smaller and harder to come by. I routinely see women traveling an hour or more to seek quality, out-of-hospital care. I'm sure that pales in comparison to some communities.

If a free-standing birth center or a licensed home-birth midwife is not available in your area and travel isn't an option, use the questions above to find a practitioner (OB or CNM or even a Family Physician) who will support you in your quest for a birth with minimal intervention.

The moral of the story is that you need to choose the people you will have around you during labor with care. You should not have to try to convince your support team that you are capable of giving birth, while in labor. A little time and energy in advance will save you a lot of grief and unnecessary communication as you labor.

In summary, yes, you have a lot of work to do to prepare yourself physically, mentally, and emotionally for this amazing, life-changing event. The time to answer all these questions has arrived, and doing it will allow you to practice the art of breathing and relaxation. Answering these questions now, while practicing relaxation daily will prepare you so that in the final days and weeks of your pregnancy, as your list of things to think about dwindles and a real birth plan begins to emerge, the breathing and relaxing will become more and more natural, even effortless. Don't worry, just breathe and relax, it takes place little-by-little, it is going to take shape over the course of the next several weeks. All you have to think about right now is your homework!

Homework for Lesson 3

See Classroom Resources on www.ExpectingKindness.com for
Reading assignments
Articles/additional resources
Links to video's
Exercise assignments
Journaling prompts
Tools for partners
Relaxation Techniques

Important tip:
Turn off phones, or at least silence the ringers and text message alert. If the phone is set to vibrate, place it on a soft surface so the aggravation of its buzzing is lessened.

Lesson 4

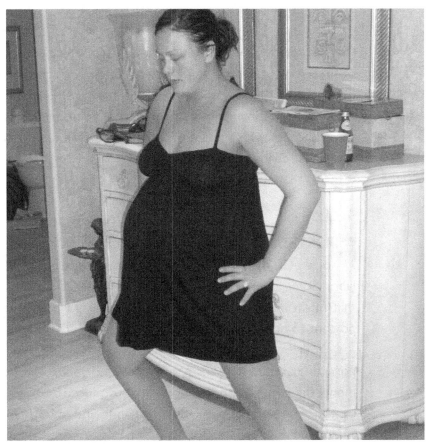

Life Actually Photography

"This was an initiation, through which I experienced a profound kinship with all women throughout history who had ever gone through this ordeal and transformation. There was nothing that distinguished me from any woman who had ever given birth to a baby"

—Jean Shinoda Bolen (b. 1936), American analyst, educator and writer

First Stage Labor

IN THIS LESSON, we are going hold a magnifying glass to the phases of first stage labor. I'll guide you through what an uncomplicated first stage of labor looks, feels, and acts like. Even though some women move through this stage faster than others, the signs, symptoms and behaviors are not really any different in a faster labor; things just change faster.

The last weeks of pregnancy

FIRST LET'S DISCUSS a few things that go on during the last days or weeks of your pregnancy that are preparatory for first stage labor. Some of this preparatory work will have physical symptoms that might make you think you are beginning labor, so they are important to understand.

Your body begins to produce certain hormones in higher than normal quantities. Oxytocin is the love hormone, the bonding hormone, the contraction hormone. It is produced as a result of physical touch, eye contact, sex, holding hands, and in both you and your baby's bodies in preparation for labor. It is responsible for your labor contractions. Rising levels of this hormone in the weeks leading up to your labor causes an increase in the Braxton Hicks (pre-labor) contractions that strengthen your uterus for its upcoming marathon. Having some contractions can indicate labor, but often women experience bouts of contractions in preparation. The normal rise in Oxytocin can also make you more emotionally raw and more sensitive.

Prolactin is another hormone that is increasing at this time. It is involved in the production of colostrum and breast milk and is also known for its "sense of calm in the face of chaos" properties. As a result, you may notice a bit of fluid, almost golden, beading from the nipple. Your body will also be "lubing the pipes" meaning your mucous membranes (the birth canal being one of them) will increase production. You may notice that you are congested, and you may notice a mucous discharge coming out of the vagina.

Some women will have a little bit of cervical change prior to the onset of labor contractions. This slight dilation and/or effacement of the cervix can result in a little blood in the mucous discharge. We might call it "pink tinged mucous." As the cervix opens, little capillaries rupture (you don't feel it). If you have bleeding more than "pink tinged mucous" it can still be very normal, but it's best to let your birth team be the judge; they'll want to be aware of any cervical change anyway.

Your birth team may have a specific list of reasons to make contact with them, make sure you know what they want you to communicate and follow your birth team's protocol in these cases.

Early First Stage Labor

AS WE DISCUSSED in the brief overview in lesson 1, the entire function of first stage is to open the cervix. The first question you ask when you have some contractions is "Am I in labor?" the honest answer is that you won't know at first. It will take some time to watch for change. In the very early stages of labor, there is little to no cervical dilation and therefore the signs and symptoms will be very subtle. I am a big believer in only giving your labor the attention it is demanding, so at this stage I recommend practically ignoring it. A few contractions here or there shouldn't limit your activity except in these few circumstances.

1. If you are far away from your home or desired birth location, use (potential) early labor as a reason to mobilize.
2. If your partner is at work, away on business or away from you, it's time to make the call. Come home.

"Am I in labor?"

You will tell the story of this day a thousand times and remember it for the rest of your life.

3.   If it is during a time of night when you would normally be sleeping, try to ignore it altogether and see if you can get a few hours of sleep collected between contractions.

Otherwise, treat your early labor like a dress rehearsal, as it sometimes is, and act like it's a nice, relaxed Saturday. Be really kind to yourself, be restful, have some tea, go to a movie, take a walk, read, crochet, or whatever makes you feel calm and relaxed. Welcome the contractions. Avoid startling your sphincters! Let your labor gain traction. Try to make good memories; you will tell the story of this day a thousand times and remember it for the rest of your life. I can't emphasize enough about accumulating rest/sleep at this time. I have a lot of women tell me that that feel like, or think that, they will have a fast labor...or an early labor...but statistics tell another story. Most first time Mama's will go beyond their estimated due date and labor for roughly 18-24 hours. Plan for that...laugh at me later! Prepare for the challenge and then be happy if it's sooner (hopefully not too soon) or faster (hopefully not too fast) than expected.

Once your contractions become more regular, you can time them periodically to see if there is a change, but again, don't give it more attention than it requires. This phase is one of the biggest time variables; some women kick right into a regular labor pattern while others hover here for quite some time. You might even venture into "prodromal labor," a longer than normal early phase that sometimes takes days, to "turn over." No matter which way your labor goes, being careful to rest whenever possible and conserve your energy could prove very valuable if moves slowly or starts and stops, and starts and stops again. Here are some things you may notice throughout this early phase.

- The feeling that "This could be it!" Something is happening! It is exciting, no doubt. This isn't really the time to call everyone in your address book or share on social media. You don't how long your labor will last and you can cause needless worry and put yourself at risk of receiving incessant phone calls and texts from loved ones if they know too soon. I suggest waiting a while to see if things progress.

- An obsessive need to "do something" in preparation for the baby. I call this "power-nesting" and it can range from washing and folding the baby's clothes to shampooing the carpets or cleaning out the refrigerator. Generally, it's just an outlet for nervous, excited energy, directed toward preparing for baby.

- Contractions may be as far apart as thirty minutes or more, or as close as five or ten minutes. They usually are relatively short, lasting twenty to forty-five seconds.

- You may feel contractions in the lower back, low in the abdomen, like menstrual cramps, or starting in one area and wrapping around the belly. Many women can talk and/or walk right straight through these early contractions, or perhaps just pause for breath at the peak for a few seconds and then resume the conversation or activity they were engaged in before it started.

- When you are not resting, or trying to accumulate moments of sleep between contractions, being active can be helpful

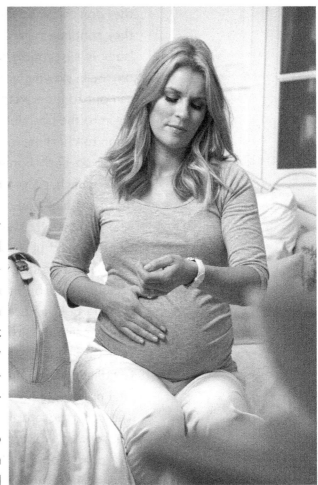

during this stage of labor. It is common knowledge that women who are changing positions frequently through first stage labor—moving and listening to the cues the body offers—often progress through first stage faster than sedentary women.

Arriving at your birth place too early.

IF YOU HAVE had a healthy prenatal course and there are no specific concerns, it is usually in your best interest to avoid checking in at your birthplace if you are less than 5cm dilated. Your birth team will tell you if there are specific concerns that would require you to go in sooner than later. At approximately five centimeters, you cross a threshold into active first stage labor. Contractions are generally very regular and don't change in response to a car ride, they don't slow down when a few unfamiliar people enter the room, they continue regardless of position. Prior to five centimeters your labor is susceptible to stress/excitement, as adrenaline can usurp oxytocin, slowing and sometimes even stopping contractions. You can opt to meet your doctor at his or her office instead of checking in to the hospital or ask to be examined in triage at the hospital prior to checking in. If you are less than five centimeters, you can either go back home, go to a local park, go to nearby hotel, go out to lunch, go get a pedicure, a massage, go visit a friend; pretty much anything you consider normal and comfortable will help your labor progress faster than having exams every hour or two and being hooked up to machines while people stare at you. Intensive watchfulness can sometimes increase the risk of intervention. The pressure to progress is often palpable, even if it is only perceived, and the policies driving staff to take over and manage your labor can be painfully obvious. Treat this situation the same regardless of your care provider. Even if you are lucky enough to have access to a Certified Nurse Midwife in the hospital, they are still bound by hospital policy and procedure, and can only work with you to a point. The other potential variable is the nursing staff. There are nurses who opt to work in obstetrics for all the right reasons, they are passionate about childbirth, they have a gift for caring for women during labor, they have incredibly relevant experience that makes them an unbelievable caregiver. But there are others. The others work in obstetrics because it is the shift they needed, or they like babies, or they don't really have a preference. Some began as example one, but over a period of years, have become de-sensitized to the individual woman because we all blend together after 1000 births. I have heard them in the halls complaining about women who vocalize, women who have birth plans, women who are "difficult" (meaning informed), women who have opinions about their care, women who ask too many questions. Arriving too early to the hospital is one of the biggest reasons for the rate of intervention up to and including cesarean section. There are nurses that will be patient and supportive, but we can't guarantee that we will get that nurse, so laboring at home until you actively need what the hospital offers is a safer bet.

Don't check in too early and be subjected to "pressure to progress." Arrive when there is work to be done.

Arriving early at a freestanding birth center is less risky as far as forced intervention, but not terribly different when you consider that even watchful observation, taking your blood pressure, temperature and listening to the baby and checking the cervix intermittently (which is likely to be protocol) is still both distracting and stimulating, not really conducive to calm, steady, progress. Early in the dilation process, just being aware of and feeling observed can stifle your labor progress. Not often talked about, is the idea of going home again after arriving at your birth center. It is fairly common for women in labor to arrive earlier than is ideal, the reason being that labor feels pretty hard, harder than you'd think, before there is a need to be at the birthplace. In an Out Of Hospital birth, there is an additional concern, OOH midwives don't have daily shifts the way in hospital staff does. They are often on call for a week, then off for a week or two, then on again. We need your midwife to be as sharp as a tac at the time of birth, when all their knowledge and skills are most needed. Spending hours and hours and hours with you as you move into and through much of your active labor is the job of the Doula, or your close family or friends. There are exceptions, reasons you may need to have them closer to you, but I recommend trusting their guidance. If they are encouraging you to go home, it is because they believe that you will make more progress there.

The extent of my research on this topic is admittedly limited by my experiences and geography, but does span hundreds of births and many hospitals, birth centers, and home births in a "progressive" region. I will not list specific experiences to drive the point home, but will strongly encourage you to arrive when there is work to be done and when you actively need, not want, what your birthplace and staff has to offer you. Wanting to need to be there and needing to be there are not always the same thing.

> Active first stage labor isn't subtle. You'll know.

Active First Stage Labor

THE GREAT THING about active first stage labor is that you won't be wondering, "Is this it?" It isn't subtle. As you progress further into your labor, there are some predictable changes in how you communicate, move, and behave. This changes the support you need, the positions you find comfortable, your breathing, and so on. This phase is a good time to begin to communicate with your birth team if you haven't made contact already.

- Emotionally you may feel a sense of acceptance, like, "Oh, ok. This is what labor feels like." You may begin to get a sense of the work that contractions bring, but assuming you have had some rest and that you have a good understanding of what is happening, you will likely still feel strong, empowered, and not overwhelmed by these sensations.

- Many women in this stage of labor are still taking a walk close to home, eating regular meals, and functioning relatively normally with the exception of needing to stop to breathe through more of - if not all of - the contraction, now approximately sixty seconds.

- You will probably begin to see a solid contraction pattern emerge; they become somewhat predictable. Contractions that are roughly five minutes apart for a period of about an hour, last close to sixty seconds, and don't change in frequency if you change your activity—eat a meal, drink some water, walk around—or change your environment are a great sign that your labor is making progress and that it is becoming active.

- You may find that a routine for coping with contractions becomes important. Certain positions, certain touch, certain words and/or slow, deep breathing can provide a rhythm and comfort you.

- You may begin to feel more pain or pressure in your lower back, the bones of the pelvis begin to ache as the baby begins to descend and the ligaments and muscles that are connected to the pelvis stretch and ache. These are great signs that your body is doing what it needs to do to allow the baby to begin to descend. Think of the discomfort as a map, telling you where your baby is, reassuring you that this choreographed dance is moving your baby.

- At this point, you (or your partner) should time your contractions over the course of an hour. Make a note of how far apart they are and how long they are lasting to report to your birth team the next time you check in. Yes, there is an app for that.

Avoid apps that tell you what stage of labor you are in based on contractions alone, it is more complicated than that.

- Because of the increased intensity and frequency of contractions in addition to the added sensations of the baby's descent, you may need a little more support. It is best if your birth partner can be with you from this point forward, if you do not have a birth partner available and have hired a labor doula, this is the right time contact her and request her presence. Labor can take a while from this point to birth, or it can move quite swiftly, but either way you are ready for additional support. If you have opted to not hire a labor doula, have someone— best friend, sister, mother, mother-in-law, niece, etc.—on call to come and help if labor becomes more challenging or longer than your primary partner can handle alone. You will not enjoy being left alone as labor progresses from here, and your partner may need to eat, rest, or use a bathroom once in a while. Remember that *your* body is functioning like an athlete, bordering on superhuman, with endorphins coursing through your veins. Your partner is just a normal human being and susceptible to normal bodily needs and functions.

When your contractions are less than five minutes apart and lasting more than sixty seconds, you should communicate with your birth team.

There is some ambiguity between the early first stage of labor and the beginning of this active phase. Look for the cues listed above and identify emerging patterns and emotional/physical needs and changes. A woman in this stage may need some pressure on her back as the strength of the contractions peak, pulling harder on those pelvic bones, joints and ligaments. She may be realizing that the power and intensity her uterus is capable of is more than she expected. She may need to be reminded why she is feeling what she is feeling. The uterus is a powerful muscle, stronger contractions are good sign that work is being done. She may express frustration if her partner is not in the right place when the contraction kicks in, or is not pushing in the right spot at the right time. She may become irritated if her partner's attention is divided. All of these are great signs so don't become discouraged or offended by any criticism; smile on the inside, it's working!

The visibly progressing active phase is usually easy to identify, and it is the most important one to recognize because it is the

The two parts of our bodies that we have been required to cover since we were little girls are the very two parts that are needed to get the baby in there, and to get the baby out and provide immediate care.

catalyst for making the move to your birth center/hospital or asking your midwifery team to join you at home.

When your contractions are less than five minutes apart and lasting more than sixty seconds, you should communicate with your birth team. They will probably ask you to come in. It may still be wise to get checked prior to making the commitment of checking in to the hospital or birth center. If you choose to verify dilation, have your exam even before the emotional commitment of bringing all the bags in. If you follow these guidelines, you will hopefully arrive at the right time. If you are checked and discover that you still have some time, go back home, take a shower, and continue with your comfort tools and continuous support. Watch for the specific changes offered by your care provider, try to rest and relax between contractions.

If your cervix is dilated to five centimeters or more, it is time to get comfy, check in, get bags, or keep your midwifery team at your side. Here comes the roller coaster.

Occasionally, the act of checking in at your birth place can cause a little lull in contractions. Just get comfortable in the new environment and they normally resume.

- First, a climb. From the point where contractions are lasting over a minute and are as frequent as three to five minutes apart you are really working hard. Your attitude is focused, you concentrate on your slow deep abdominal breathing to get through the peak of the contraction, which is now lasting somewhere in the thirty-second range and has grown in intensity to demand all of your attention.
- Most women dislike being distracted from their focus and will give "feedback" freely if focus is disrupted.
- Another fun symptom of this phase of labor is the loss of modesty. This doesn't mean that your modest self will all of a sudden become an exhibitionist; it's actually quite the opposite. You will likely be entirely unconcerned with how your nudity, or partial nudity, may affect those around you. It is an animal instinct when you boil it down. The two parts of our bodies that we have been required to cover since we were little girls are the very two parts that are often needed to get the baby

in there, and also to get the baby out and provide immediate care and contact. In its ancient wisdom, your body knows this.

- Additionally, women at this stage of labor have swings in body temperature, working as hard as a mountain climber and sweating during contractions, then chilling between contractions as the heat from exertion recedes and the sweat cools the skin. It is much easier to regulate these swings if we don't have clothes on; pulling up a blanket between and flinging it off as contractions begin is just easier. Many women also feel that clothing feels binding and adds to the pressure and discomfort.

- You may feel the need to vocalize. This is somewhat related to the loss of modesty in so far as most non-laboring people would try to avoid public moaning if possible. If done correctly, vocalization can be very helpful for two reasons. First, it feels better. Little children moan when they don't feel good; it's instinctive. Second, moaning is conducive to relaxation. Low tones facilitate the descent of the baby. The alternative—shrieking and squealing—tightens the muscles making passage through the pelvis, pubococcygeus (kegel) muscle and birth canal difficult. There are some women who are virtually silent, which is also just fine. The only symptom of their being awake is the increase in the rate and depth of breathing during contractions.

- Nausea—good times. It appears to me to be caused by a combination of the rise in body temperature during contractions along with significant pressure on the cervix or cervical change. Nausea can be magnified by putting anything in the tummy, but staying hydrated trumps nausea and if you do end up gagging/vomiting, having water is better than being dry. Most women feel at least a little nausea sometime between this point and the shift to pushing.

During this climbing phase of first stage, there are specific tasks, tools and techniques that can have a huge effect on how Mom handles the contractions and the changes happening, or alternately, handling the contractions during a longer labor pattern with a lack of significant change. So, from here we diverge into two labor scenarios:

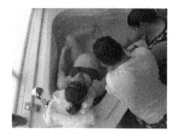

Scenario A
Active first stage labor with obvious cervical change

IF YOU HAVE been examined upon arrival and are dilated 5 centimeters or more and your cervix is showing change, OR my personal favorite, we arrive when there is no question about whether or not it's time to be there and the tub is filled and waiting for her to get in, now we can focus entirely on your physical comfort and allow your body to do the work. Changing positions occasionally is still beneficial. Depending on what you have available at your birth place, you may try some of the following:

Take fifteen to thirty minutes in any of the following positions, in any order:

Tub

Even if your provider won't let you deliver in the tub, laboring in one takes a whole level of intensity away. They call it the natural epidural for a very good reason. If you are willing to move around and get into different positions in the tub you are more likely to make continued progress and can stay in longer, getting out periodically to pee, stretch out, or move around. In or out of the tub, changing position often can help your baby move through the pelvis. Some positions that many women will intuitively use are; hands and knees, sitting upright, slightly reclined, squatting, standing, swaying, leaning on an exercise ball, side lying. You can do all of these, some with slight variations in the tub. I do recommend saving the tub for the big guns, waiting until you are in really active labor when it will have its most profound effect. If you've been in the tub for hours, it won't seem like such a dramatic change.

Some care providers don't push, or even offer the tub because it makes their job a little harder. For example, nurses and doctors I have worked with almost universally don't like to or won't "check you"—pelvic exam to determine dilation—in the tub. Ironically, that's a great reason to be in there. It is sort of a pain if you are attached to all the hospital bells and whistles—external fetal monitor, I.V., blood pressure monitor, etc.—to get everything hooked up in the bathroom. Do what you can to minimize your leashes and really push for laboring through late first stage and transition with the tub available to you.

Toilet

I love the toilet during labor. You should really be drinking enough water during this stage to require a pit stop every hour or so anyway. Time and time again, I have seen women make amazing progress sitting on the toilet. Why? We have been trained since early childhood to relax the kegel muscle while perched there. It is involuntary, and very often extremely effective. Keeping your bladder empty is critically important, too. When full, it acts as a barrier that your baby has to push past. Keeping the path unobstructed is the best plan. Every hour or so, spend five to fifteen minutes hanging out on the toilet. You can sit backwards, leaning onto the tank, or onto some pillows if that is more comfortable. This position can also give your support team full access to your back, arms and legs for massage.

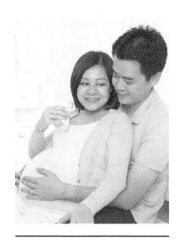

You should be drinking enough water to require a pit stop every hour!

Walk/Dance/Sway

You are unlikely to cover too much distance at this point, but some women feel a strong sense of control and power if they stay upright and somewhat active. For five to fifteen minutes, lean against a partner, a counter, or kneel during contractions, but stay upright and active in between. This encourages the baby's descent through the use of gravity, combined with the movement of the hips and an open stance.

Rest

Rest positions interspersed with active or challenging positions for five to fifteen minutes at a time can give us the opportunity to evaluate changes since the last rest. Are the contractions stronger? Longer? Are there changing sensations, etc.? This is also an opportunity to rest those active muscle groups.

You can be restful in a variety of positions: Forward leaning over a birth ball or sofa or bed, side lying on a bed, a sofa, the floor, even on a blanket on the grass. The tub, if available, can be particularly wonderful as long as it doesn't slow down the contraction pattern. There are even massage pillows that have a hole in the center for the belly so you can rest fully flat on your stomach, giving your support team full access to guide the tension out of your body.

Scenario B
Active labor with slow cervical change

THIS IS THE single most common reason for intervention and it can boil down to a few simple factors, impatience being number one. I call it "Care Provider Distress." If you can verify that there are no clear warning signs that would indicate an actual medical complication, you carefully talk through concerns that your care provider may have, and there is no immediate or real maternal distress or fetal distress, you have the right to carry on with your labor and let your body work at its own pace. Care provider concerns often begin "This can indicate…" or "Statistically, women who don't dilate at a rate of…" or any variation on the theme of risks that "could happen" but are not actually happening at the moment. This is not a race to the finish line.

Once you are past five centimeters, however, seeing a strong labor pattern with long, frequent contractions and many of the emotional and behavioral characteristics discussed above, but limited progress, may mean a few changes should be made in the strategy. Our goal is to spend as little time in labor as possible. Positions that "feel good" tend to feel that way because they minimize pressure—not really the goal at this point. Use all the positions and strategies in scenario A, but increase the rest periods since you will probably be less excited about doing a lot of moving and changing. A good coach will remind you that your goal is to move through your labor as efficiently as possible so you don't have to have any more contractions than are absolutely necessary. When the cervix is slower to demonstrate change, other factors that become important are related to your physical endurance. it is important to conserve energy, maintain hydration, perhaps force some nutrition, and rest periodically. If there is one thing that is universally true in labor and birth, this is it: You are capable of *far* more than you realize. I promise you that. There may be a point in a long, slow, labor where we must choose some intervention to try to avoid surgery. We will discuss informed consent in greater detail later, but suffice it to say, technology is not our enemy. We just need to be informed and make wise choices, and use technology and intervention as a last resort as much as possible, whenever the risk of intervening exceeds the risk of waiting. It's not always a clear-cut choice, there may be some gray area to navigate.

Vaginal Exams

If cervical exams are being done, it is important that a laboring woman gets credit for any cervical change. Some care providers are highly focused on dilation alone. You get credit if: the cervix is thinner (effacement), softer or ripened, has moved forward from posterior to anterior, increased dilation, baby is lower (station). If you have a provider that is stingy with positive feedback and/or is checking you too frequently to make any significant change, you do not have to let them in there. I have seen labors where someone, a nurse, midwife, doctor, sometimes a different person is trying to get up in there every thirty minutes…easily every hour. Why? I don't have the faintest idea. Boredom is my best guess. They see it as normal. They do it every day and may have forgotten that the general population does not have virtual strangers putting a hand up their vagina as part of our daily routine. Brush teeth, wash face, vaginal exam, floss… Um, No.

As a general rule, a maximum of two vaginal exams are necessary during labor. The first we have already discussed—upon arrival at your birth location to verify that you have not arrived too soon. The second would be appropriate when you feel a strong urge to push, to verify that you aren't pushing against an incomplete cervix. Other than those two, exams are stressful, often occurring far too frequently for your muscles and cervix to relax again and make progress. Imagine trying to let down and poop during a rectal examination, sounds crazy, right. It's literally exactly the same.

Ladies, have you ever had the following conversation with your Gynecologist?

Gyn: Ok, I am now going to do the internal pelvic exam, please just rest your feet in the stirrups and let your legs relax and lob out.

Woman: Yeah, ok.

Gyn: I need you to relax your legs and let your knees lob outward.

Woman: Yup.

> You do not have to let them in there.

Gyn: I mean really relax, just let your knees open nice and wide.
Woman: Oh, yeah. Ok.
Gyn: I am now going to insert the speculum, please relax your legs and let them remain open nice and wide.
Woman: Oh, right. Ok.
Gyn: You need to relax your bottom and let your legs just fall open at the knees.
Woman: Yes. Ok.

You get the point. Stressful situations have this effect, things tighten up.

If the bag of fluid is ruptured, frequent exams also increase the risk of infection due to introduced bacteria—one of the risks that are increased in a hospital environment due to the presence of "super germs" that have grown resistant to antibiotics. If the bag is unruptured, frequent exams increase the risk of artificial rupture and thus increase the risk of having a time limit imposed on your labor. That increases the risk of infection and the need for IV antibiotics. Additionally, there is often more than one care provider wanting to check you; the nurse that relieves your assigned nurse for lunch, for example. This adds the risk of differing opinions, which can be emotionally upsetting, and also requiring an additional check for the deciding vote. Above all, the reason to avoid frequent pelvic exams is… it is rarely beneficial. I have supported women who have dilated from one to ten centimeters and deliver in less than two hours. Conversely, I have supported women who labor for days and dilate slow and steady.

The question that must be answered is: If you are dilated four centimeters, what does that mean? It means that you are probably in labor, and not much more. It literally means than depending on a variety of factors, it could be a couple hours, or a day, sometimes more. It doesn't really foretell anything. Some practitioners use textbooks and statistics to define labor. Are you a textbook or a statistic? Me neither. Additionally, most women, no matter how logical, play some crazy mind games with themselves during labor. Here is the basic issue. No woman really wants to believe that she will have to work a lot harder than she is currently working. Even if she logically knows that her contractions are twenty minutes apart and only lasting forty seconds, if a vaginal exam is done, somewhere in the back of her mind she is thinking, "Please say ten centimeters, please say ten centimeters, please say ten centimeters." So, for most of your labor, the part where you are cognizant of what those words actually mean, you are likely to be disappointed every time. You want to hear "Ten." You want to hear, "Wow! You can push." You want to hear, "Here comes the baby!" Anything less is disheartening.

Remember that your provider doesn't have the right to touch you without your permission

Making Exceptions:

If you have a care provider who is seeking specific information to guide you and help you work with your body. For example: If the baby's position is preventing the descent, he or she may suggest certain positions or activities, like side lying or lunging. Remember that your provider doesn't have the right to touch you without your permission. Having an "exit only" policy forces your providers to seek your informed consent. I don't mean to imply that you should decline care without cause. I only mean that it is still your body, and if there is no obvious medical need to have uncomfortable, invasive, stressful exam while simultaneously trying to cope with contractions, don't let anyone bully you into interventions that are not medically necessary, including vaginal exams. Make them present you with a case that convinces you that it is medically indicated, that they are seeking specific information and then ask them what decisions will be made based on the data received. THEN decide if you want them to do the exam.

Summary

THE FIRST STAGE of labor has some ambiguity, to a point. After that point, it has specific challenges depending on the rate of progress. In either case it can be relaxed, hard work, fun, calm, boring, frustrating, empowering, active, endearing, defining. When you list it out like that, it's easy to see the analogy that the inventor of this process intended. All those words will be applied to parenting—sometimes literally—every day. Focus on the purpose of any discomfort, using the contractions to their fullest possible advantage and conserving your energy between contractions as we are watching and waiting for a specific set of game-changing behaviors and symptoms, which we will cover in detail in the next chapter. At this point, we simply have to make every contraction as efficient as we possibly can, so that we are facilitating change, progress.

You don't want to have one single contraction above what is really necessary. If you think about it like that, ringing every ounce of progress out of each contraction, you can choose to feel empowered—a sense of control at a time when many women feel afraid, helpless, and powerless. Use the labor, choose to internalize the strength, and let it be your strength, instead of feeling like it is happening to you. All this power and strength is radiating from your body, it is you, stronger than you knew.

Why do I feel the desire to roar right now?

I hope you feel it too.

Homework for Lesson 4

See Classroom Resources on _www.ExpectingKindness.com_ for
Reading assignments
Articles/additional resources
Links to video's
Exercise assignments
Journaling prompts
Tools for partners
Relaxation techniques

Lesson 5

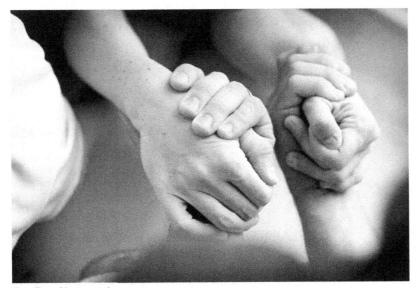

One Tree Photography

Help us to be ever faithful gardeners of the spirit, who know that without darkness nothing comes to birth, and without light nothing flowers.

May Sarton

Transition

LIKE THE OTHER stages discussed in previous lessons, I am going over the typical, uncomplicated birth process here. Any questions you have regarding "what ifs" will be addressed while we are working on writing your detailed birth plan and preparing for any possible detours from your intended experience.

Let's just take the rest of this one little step at a time, just like real labor.

Transition

AS EXPLAINED IN the overview, transition is literally changing gears between first and second stage labor. What is actually happening is this: the strong first stage contraction pattern continues, pulling and holding the cervix open. These contractions are rising and falling (still a wave-like sensation, but longer, and with higher, longer peaks) every two to three minutes and lasting over a minute, sometimes lasting as long as ninety seconds. Then, these new contractions, "pushing contractions" begin to press down, moving the baby down through the cervix, filling that space.

The net result is that for a period of time the labor is hard and unpredictable. In first stage labor, we knew what to expect and so it was easier, even when it was hard. In transition, the contractions aren't necessarily harder, but not knowing when the contraction will come makes it feel harder. For most women, this is the most challenging part of labor for a variety of reasons.

Emotionally, it is hard to even know what you are feeling. Feeling out of control is normal. Mentally, it is very challenging because your ability to be rational, think clearly, and articulate what you need is somewhat impaired. It takes all of your focus to relax and breathe through contractions and prepare for the next one while using your little break to the fullest. Physically, it is truly a roller coaster ride, and you can't get off. The beauty in transition is obvious to those witnessing it and often to women who have photography or videography and can look at it later and see themselves through a different lens. Transition is beautiful because you really get to see how powerful your body is, and because is it usually the shortest of all the stages of labor, generally only lasting fifteen to thirty minutes. So, yeah, it's tough, but it is a finite amount of time that you have to commit to really toughing it out.

It's tough, but it is a finite amount of time that you have to commit to really toughing it out.

This is the point in labor in which most women will ask for relief in some form. It may be as simple as needing a hand to hold or pressure in the right spot at the right time, every time, without exception. But we live in a society where "quick fixes" are a constant expectation. Many women ask for an epidural even if they know that it isn't an option, even if they don't really want it.

To get back to the analogy of the athlete, I invite you to imagine yourself on mile twenty of a marathon, running uphill. The finish line isn't visible yet, you can't see over the hill and you don't know what the terrain of the last six miles looks like. Is it all going to be like this? Will it be harder? Tired, thirsty, dusty, sweaty; legs, ankles, and feet aching; you glance to the left and driving next to you is a gorgeous limousine, equipped with bottled water, snacks, blankets, a nice soft place to lie down and a hand being held out. You hear a voice say "Come on, why are you doing this to yourself? You don't have to prove anything. Don't you want to just lie down?" If you get in, the last 6 miles might be a piece of cake, but there is a significantly increased risk that you could crash. Getting in has its own set of risks that many women don't consider when the hand is reaching out to them. The most important risk is this: you don't know who is driving.

It's sort of a cheap tactic, actually, offering an epidural (the limo) to a woman who is perfectly capable and in the final stretch, at her most vulnerable moment. What the voice was saying was true, you don't have to do this… you don't have anything to prove and you may actually want to get in that car, but those are not the important questions. The important questions are: Will you wonder if you could have done it? Will you wish later that you had not been offered the ride? If complications arise that change the outcome of your birth, will you be able to look back at this moment and say, I made the right decision? Will you have to harbor those unanswerable "what if" questions in the back of your mind?

Many women say things like "I can't do this" or "I give up," and sometimes a more entertaining version comes up like "I will give you my leg if you make it stop," or "I want to go home, I don't want to do this anymore." The incredibly ironic thing about these statements is that "giving up" is exactly what needs to be done, but not in the way that you might think. Let go of the idea of controlling the physical power of your body and give in to it. Let your body be powerful, let your body do the hard work. Let go. Give in. Breathe. Relax. Even more. Early first stage, and active first stage have been preparing you for this. You are almost there. Breathe slower, deeper, release more, soften your body, let go, release.

> Let go of the idea of controlling the physical power of your body and give in to it.

Physical signs and symptoms of transition

- The strength and length of contractions will cause her to perspire
- Muscle fatigue and adrenaline can cause her body to shake involuntarily
- She may feel nauseous, she may burp, she may vomit (can be a very beneficial downward thrust)
- Her extremities (hands and feet) may be cold due to the blood flow being focused on the muscles that are working the hardest
- For a short time, the contractions may simply feel like they never go away, however, over the course of the transition process the expulsive contractions will start to take over and the intense frequent contractions working hard to pull the last bit of cervix back will begin to release their grip. You may begin to hear some guttural grunts or a short burst of an involuntary

push at the peaks of some of the contractions. *These are all signs that transition
is almost over*

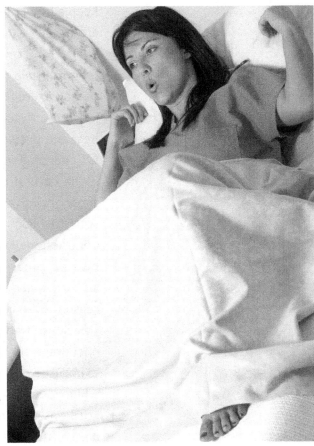

- She may express feeling "a lot of pressure" or fear that she may need to have a
bowel movement.

- She may need almost constant physical
support, constant reassurance that everything's all right, that her body is amazing and doing exactly what it is supposed
to be doing, that the baby is moving down
causing pressure and that occasional urge
to push. Some women have a hard time
believing it when we tell them that they
can listen to their bodies and give a little
push if it feels good. If it pinches or feels
wrong, a sign that a rim of cervix is still
there, continue to try to breathe through
those contractions, taking one at a time,
until the urge is uncontrollable, undeniable

- Unless it is incredibly obvious that she is complete (10cm),
most care providers will want to do an exam to make sure
the cervix is gone. I can get on board with that, pushing against
remaining cervix can cause it to swell, like a fat lip, which can
prolong transition.

Specific support and coping during transition

- She will typically *not* be ok being left alone, from this point on
someone should be vigilantly present and focused on her all
the time. It's fine to work together to make sure all her needs
are being met, if you have a large enough team.

- Cold compresses on her neck, forehead and chest and to wipe
her face can reduce her body temperature and minimize feelings of overheating and nausea. You may need to swap them
out as each contraction begins because her body temperature
will warm them up quickly. It becomes routine and quick if you

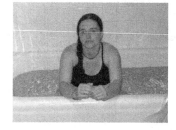

keep a bowl of ice water with a few cloths soaking while a few are in use

- Warm/hot compresses on the lower back or low on the abdomen can help to melt away tension. I have seen a few women demonstrate use of this tool so beautifully that I could literally judge the descent of the baby by watching where she needed heat and pressure.

- Of course, if you have a tub available to you, *get in!* They call it the natural epidural for good reason. For most women, it simply removes an entire layer of the intensity. The only reasons to NOT use the tub include: a swelling cervix, slowing contractions, overheating, high blood pressure/elevated heart rate or other specific medical concerns that are presented and explained thoroughly. Convenience isn't a good enough reason. Even if you don't have the option to have a water birth, you can still labor in it until you are through transition. I usually encourage the use of showers in early labor and limited tub exposure so that it can have a powerful effect in the moment when you need it most.

- Positions. Plural. Change it often but try to remain somewhat upright most of the time. I will never forget a story a midwife told me once about arriving on the scene for a homebirth, finding the mother on her knees with her booty in the air and her head on the floor. She reported that this position felt "more comfortable." Well, yes, but she was making her baby climb uphill to get out! We need gravity, good position, movement, and strong contractions.

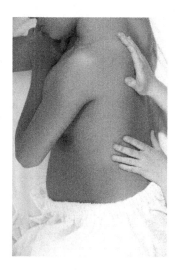

- You may walk, sway, stand, kneel, lean, lie down, squat, lunge and sit—in virtually any order! Make sure that your team can provide physical support both to stabilize you during contractions and to provide comfort.

- For massage, I personally prefer natural grape seed or comfrey infused oil. It's natural, readily available, great for your skin, and lasts a while. You can infuse it with herbs if you like or purchase fancy infusions, but be careful that it isn't too aromatic, even smells you enjoy can seem overwhelming during labor

- Tennis sized ball. You can roll it in small circles at the sacrum during contractions. I prefer the "classic pinky ball" sold commonly at drug stores in the toy aisle. Perfect foam pressure, plus it's fun to play with your baby later!

- Simple back pressure at the sacrum, supporting the bones as baby moves through the pelvis.
- Double hip squeeze, helps to open the pelvis and relieves pressure. I have only worked with one or two women that didn't really dig this one. 99% success rate.
- A Transition massage sequence: Up the ante. Rhythm is key, use music to give you some guidance if she likes it. Routine is key, she will find comfort in repetition, in constancy. For example: firm hands guiding the tension down and out of her body, beginning from the neck and shoulders and moving tension down through her arms and out gently through the fingertips, then begin again at the neck and stroke firmly down her back to the sacrum, a strong press right at the tailbone, then move the hands out to the hips and give a nice firm squeeze there, pressing in and back at the Ilium. (Image search: posterior, pelvis, ilium) Repeat as necessary until contraction ends.

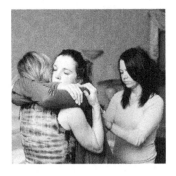

You must challenge the idea that this is something happening to you, and instead recognize that what you are experiencing is you, however involuntary.

Summary

KNOW THAT this particular stage of labor sounds hard. Yeah, well, it is hard. It is why you need to be prepared; it is the reason why it is so critical that you know that your body is capable of far more than you realize. Those moments when you don't feel like you can go on for another minute do come, and they go. And with each passing moment of perceived weakness, you begin to realize your strength. You need to surround yourself with people you can trust to hold your hand through one of the greatest defining moments of your life. You must challenge the idea that this is something happening to you, and instead recognize that what you are experiencing is you, however involuntary.

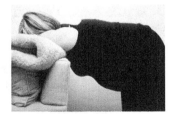

One Tree Photography

Use the contraction. Squeeze every solitary ounce of progress out of it and make it work for you. Let your body relax, let the contraction be strong, and take your brain out of the equation. I promise you, it will be over much sooner if you breathe and relax

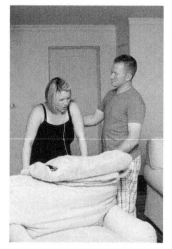

One Tree Photography

into it; fighting it makes it last longer and hurt more. Please believe me, and prepare.

One of the most interesting things about this stage of labor is how internal the chaos is. When I take photographs of women at this stage, they are always very surprised later to see that on the outside—while all of that internal physical, mental and emotional intensity was happening—she looks like she's sleeping, relaxing completely in response to the chaos. At times, we can only tell that she is having a contraction because her rate and depth of breathing increases. I cannot think of a training exercise more relevant for entering motherhood. Relax and breathe in response to chaos.

You can't argue with that!

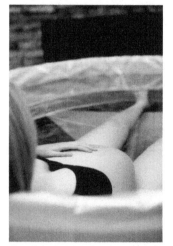

One Tree Photography

Homework for Lesson 5

See Classroom Resources on www.ExpectingKindness.com for
Reading assignments
Articles/additional resources
Links to video's
Exercise assignments
Journaling prompts
Tools for partners
Relaxation techniques

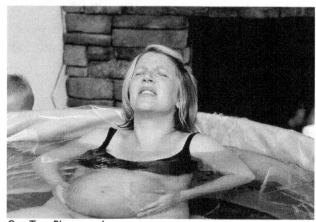

One Tree Photography

Lesson 6

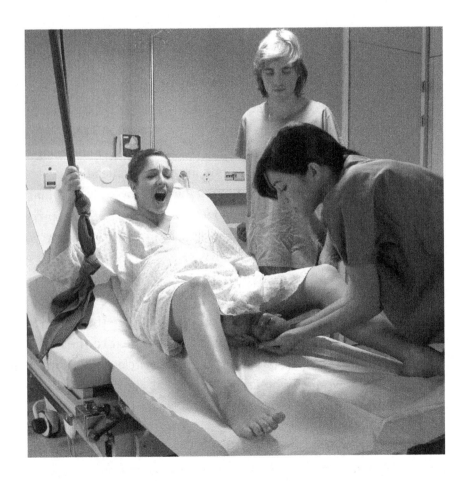

"There is no way out of the experience except through it, because it is not really your experience at all, but the baby's. Your body is the child's instrument of birth."

—Penelope Leach, British psychologist

Second Stage: Pushing

Preparation

LIKE FIRST STAGE labor there are things that happen prior to labor beginning that are in preparation for this moment. One systemic change you will have noticed is the softening of the cartilage throughout your body in the weeks leading up to your labor. Your grip weakens, and your hips feel wobbly. The function of this chemical change is to allow your pelvis to open approximately 10-20% further than it normally can in order to allow your baby to move through the pelvic basin.

Another systemic change you will notice is an evacuation of your intestinal tract. Most women will experience "loose stool" in the hours or days leading up to labor. Since the baby needs to move through the birth canal, which is right next to the rectum, the body knows that the path must be (mostly) clear. This knowledge should calm women who are concerned about having a bowel movement during labor—specifically while pushing.

Pooping

THERE IS NO subtle way to discuss this but because this fear is so common, I won't ignore it. Honest truth is, sometimes a little poo will come out while pushing. So what? First and foremost, you should know that any trained staff that you have around you absolutely doesn't care... at all. In fact, we are encouraged by it, because involuntary pooping at this point in labor means the baby is moving down. We know to expect it and now you do, too.

If it happens, you may not even know it. If you are laboring in a bed, on the floor, or on a birth stool, you will have either towels or chux pads (plastic lined absorbent pads (like puppy potty training pads) underneath you. The top pad is simply removed and you are none the wiser. You might ask, "How could I not know?" At this stage of labor there is a lot of pressure in your bottom and it is hard to tell the difference between the rectal pressure of a bowel movement and the vaginal pressure of the baby. I have worked with many women who believed they were having a bowel movement when they weren't and many others who attributed the pressure to the baby. There have been a few that kind of knew, but also felt compelled to ask, "Did I just…?"

If you are in a tub, it's not always as easy to "remove the evidence" with the above subtlety. It commonly involves a little fishy net and a savvy doula or midwife with finesse. It may sound odd right now, but in the moment, when you are really focused on your work and thinking about "being done"—when you are simply primal in so many ways—you are unlikely to really give a shit. HA! I secretly think that this is another one of nature's brilliant birth metaphors telling us, "Your new world is just one bodily function after another…get used to it There is no room for modesty in motherhood."

Ladies, if you are worried or scared that your birth partner might see this and be "grossed out," just remember that your partner poops every day and knows that you do too. It isn't that big a deal unless you make it into one. If you are exceedingly modest and afraid of this possibility, there are a few things that you can do. Eat plenty of fiber in the last weeks of your pregnancy and stay very well hydrated. If you are beyond rational at the thought and the word phobic or panic has entered your mind while reading this passage, you and your care provider could also explore the possibility of an enema during your early labor. While an enema can sometimes stimulate labor contractions in addition to evacuating any waste, you should consider whether it will really ease your fears of pooping in public.

I offer one piece of advice to expecting parents, especially if this is something that you are particularly concerned about. It

"Your new world is just one bodily function after another… get used to it."

involves an appropriate use of the "don't ask, don't tell" act. She literally never needs to know either that it happened or that you noticed. Partners, even if she asks, you can simply plead the 5th. After she has changed her 1000th diaper (which won't take as long as you might think) and her focus is shifted to other bodily functions: baby poo/pee, breastfeeding, sleeping for more than 20 minutes at a time, it won't be an issue anymore. Motherhood has a way of disarming modesty.

Pushing

So NOW WE have arrived at the pushing (2nd) stage with relaxed cartilage in your pelvis (and everywhere else) and a mostly clear path. Your transition, what most women would consider the hardest part, is over and you are left with the contractions that press downward to expel the baby. Welcome to the most misunderstood stage of labor. This is the stage that we see in movies, sitcoms, and medical shows demonstrated by women screaming and flailing (either comically or tragically depending on the genre) with no respite, no rest, seemingly in constant and unbearable pain. Even video's and television programs designed to "educate," edit out the boring downtime in between contractions, giving the illusion that it looks like she is contracting and pushing all the time.

The shift to second stage is a relief for most women I have worked with and interviewed. It is even described as exciting, especially if mom is well supported and has a team that gives this moment the appropriate reverence. This is what we have been waiting around for—what every contraction that has been breathed through, relaxed through, and toughed out has been leading up to. The whole first stage and all the challenges of transition, have been building up to this very moment when someone finally says some variation of this statement:

"You are complete. You can push with your next contraction."

When you are well supported by an experienced team, the mood in the room changes and excitement builds. As a Doula, I am usually inspired in this moment to let out a big (whispered) "YES!" or a happy dance, even if it is invisible to Mama. The contrast from transition alone makes it seem like a breath of fresh air and

> The whole first stage and all the challenges of transition, have been building up to this very moment

the breaks between contractions are long enough for casual conversation, reflecting on your experience so far, jokes, laughter, and sometimes even quick little naps or snacks. There are even periods of boredom in many labors where women are anxiously awaiting the next contraction so they can be done faster. The contractions do come but they feel completely different from the overwhelming strength, length and intensity of the transitional contraction. The pushing response, which is often largely involuntary, is also a means of pain control. It feels good to push, right up until the point of crowning. We'll get to that.

If we are wise, we acknowledge that this isn't the finish line, and there are still some variables that can come up, but in the scheme of an uncomplicated birth, this is a major milestone and it should be celebrated as such.

As the baby descends into the birth canal, you will feel an undeniable increase in pressure, of course. Knowing to expect this pressure is very important. It is often surprising, and can make the pushing process take much longer if the doctor, midwife or doula has to continuously remind a laboring woman that the pressure is what we want; it is what brings the baby down and out. The only remotely relevant experience we have to compare this pressure to is having a bowel movement. It is physiologically about identical, except for the size of what… or who (not sure about the grammar rules when comparing a bowel movement to a tiny human being) is being evacuated.

As the baby moves through the cervix and into the birth/vaginal canal, the baby's head begins to create pressure (through the tissue separating them) on the rectal wall, creating that familiar urge to "bear down." Of course, the baby is quite a bit larger than your average bowel movement, and causes more pressure, which causes a greater urge to push.

"How do I push?" you may be wondering. The best answer is that you don't have to work too hard to learn this particular skill because it is largely involuntary. Some practice prior to labor will allow you to get into a rhythm faster and get to the good stuff. So, if you want to keep with the "efficiency model," making the most of each contraction, follow these instructions:

The Art of Pushing

THERE ARE MANY ideas about how a woman should push. One of the beauties of having an unmedicated labor and birth is that you are free to choose what position to push in and you have the sensations to guide you in your pushing. Some women choose to work with their bodies by just breathing through most of this stage; allowing the baby to "labor down." This means to allow your uterus to do the work of moving the baby down until an uncontrollable urge to push presents itself. As long as progress is being made and there are no risks to Mom or baby, it is perfectly safe to allow a woman in this stage to simply listen to what her body is telling her to do. There is no rush. Well, except for the fact that she probably doesn't really desire to push for hours and hours and would probably prefer to be done with labor and be holding her baby. Some women have a powerful urge to bear down and push with contractions right away and must work with their bodies by actively pushing. The act of pushing is simply a combination of position and breath holding, which is somewhat instinctive, but with some focus on physiology and timing, we can make each push, each contraction as effective as possible. Below you will find a description of the most efficient pushing technique, in my opinion. This pushing technique can be applied in any position. As you practice, please use a mock breath holding technique, close your mouth and breathe through your nose. Practice will help you develop your rhythm faster during labor, shortening the second stage and putting your baby in your arms as soon as possible.

As the contraction begins, you take deep, slow, breaths. Start with the abdomen and continue in a wave like motion filling your lungs.

Breathe in through your nose and breathe out through your mouth.

1. Inhale ~ Exhale (a full yogic breath cycle)
2. Inhale ~ Exhale (two is ok if your urge to push is undeniable)
3. Inhale ~ As you begin your third breath, pull yourself into your chosen position.

No matter which position you choose, you will need to do four things as you hold your breath to make your push as efficient as possible.

Relax completely between contractions and breathe deeply to save your energy.

    A.   Curl or tilt your pelvis forward, as if you are trying to see the baby's head.

    B.   Put your chin on your chest, curling your body around your baby like the letter C.

    C.   Do your best to not release any air, <u>close your throat tight</u> and press down, while curling forward.

    D.   Hold for as close to ten seconds as you can. Exhale.

You can usually get two or three strong, (approximately) 10-second-long, pushes within each contraction so follow these steps until contraction releases. After your strong, long push, release the breath through your mouth (faster), and take in another deep breath, and go again, wringing every ounce of power out of each contraction will bring your baby into your arms sooner.

Relax completely between contractions and breathe deeply to save your energy for the next powerful contraction and effective push. Using this deep abdominal (yogic) breath does aid in effective pushing, both because of the added intra-abdominal pressure and the fact that your muscles, your body, and every cell, function better when oxygenated. You and your baby have this in common. When you breathe slowly and deeply between contractions you bolster the oxygen being transferred to your baby through the placenta, this is important because when the uterus tightens during a contraction, the transfer of oxygen is diminished. Your baby's heart rate will drop slightly (normal) in response but will tolerate the contraction better if you concentrate on oxygen delivery using deep yogic breath during and between contractions. It is especially important now because moving through the birth canal can cause some stress in the baby and the added oxygen is beneficial.

This technique creates a powerful chain reaction, the air in your lungs and diaphragm oxygenate your body and your baby's body and adds additional downward pressure as you curl forward, pressing down against the uterus, which is pressing down against the baby. The baby responds (as long as the head is down) by pressing back with his/her legs. You can test the theory after the birth; if you press gently on baby's feet, he/she will demonstrate the "stepping reflex".

This process of moving the baby through the birth/vaginal canal is usually a slow, gentle, and methodical process of stretching the tissue slowly and painlessly moving the baby down and out. (TV shows, movies and other media confuse effort, strength and power with pain.)

Getting through it

THERE IS AN art to pushing and while I am supportive of taking the time to get acclimated to the process, I also know that a little preparation can go a long way toward shortening the pushing stage of labor. Time limits are often imposed making risk of a Cesarean higher if pushing is "taking too long." You can get the rhythm much faster during your labor if you take a little time now, using the instructions above, and trying it out (without actually holding your breath) in a variety of positions to prepare for the variables of second stage. Like first stage, changing positions throughout the pushing stage can help the baby move through the pelvis. Remember the risks of doing continuous vaginal exams, but during this stage, if you have a practitioner that you can trust to be checking you periodically, it can be one of the exceptions because sometimes knowing the baby's position can provide good insight regarding what position(s) will be the most effective for pushing.

Women commonly push in the following positions:

(She may need physical support in some of the following positions; it is hard to push and hold yourself in certain positions at the same time. Your birth team will guide you.)

1. Reclined (seated and leaning back about 45°): As you prepare to push at the onset of the 3rd inhalation, place your hands behind the knee or on top of the knee and pull your legs up and out. This pulling opens the pelvis, forces you to curl around your body and tilt the pelvis forward and gives you a sort of traction with your push.

This is a great resting position and can be effective. The risk can be sitting on your tailbone, pressing it forward and creating an obstacle for baby to get around or push through.

Changing positions throughout the pushing stage can help the baby move through the pelvis.

2. Hands and knees: Being restful on hands and knees between contractions or leaning against a ball, bed, sofa, partner, etc., and then curling your body around the baby to push or resting back on your haunches to push. You may need some cushions under your knees. (I prefer gardening pads because they don't slip like pillows and can be used in the water as well, and then in the garden later!) Use the same technique—curling pelvis forward, chin on chest etc. It all works in virtually any position.

3. Upright Squat: This is globally accepted as the most efficient position for pushing out a baby. I have spoken to a lot of women who have an emotional reservation about this position, as if it has a stigma. Perhaps the stigma is related to the primal/animal nature of it or perhaps it is perceived as too much work in the face of the current standard of a hospital bed supporting every part of the body. No matter what the stigma is rooted in, we need to just let it go. No matter what positions you push in, you are effectively in a squat position, this one just has a few additional advantages.

Physiologically, the upright squat position (which can be supported by a birthing stool, a squat bar, a support person, leaning back against a wall, the edge of the tub, etc.) is effective for a variety of reasons. First and foremost, being in a vertical position uses gravity to your advantage. Additionally, the position of an open stance squat does two important things. It forces your pelvis to tilt forward (optimum position for the baby to move through) and the pressure on the hips from the weight of your body open the outlet of the pelvis an additional 10-15%, making more room for baby to move through. This position also shortens the distance of the birth canal.

You may find that pushing in one of the more relaxing position is effective and therefore using the energy to push in an upright squat is not necessary, but if a time limit is placed upon you, or you (or your partner) are feeling the vibe of intervention swelling in the room, this is the go to position. You can certainly use it preventatively as well! Change positions periodically, but adding this effective position to your repertoire will likely shorten second stage labor.

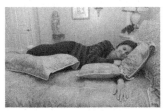

Jennifer Reif, photographer

It will take far longer to describe it than it will take for you to experience it.

---

4. Side Lying: Like all the others, you will effectively be pulling yourself into a squat position using your hands in position behind your knees and pulling your legs up and out as you bear down and curl around your baby. The advantage of this one is the ability to fully utilize the rests between contractions.

It is not uncommon to push in variety of positions, we are often moving and changing to help your baby navigate through the pelvis. Maintain that C shape, getting your body into the shape of a squat, regardless of the position you choose. Arching in response to the pressure will prolong your labor. Whether you are using breath holding, or letting your body do it, helping your baby by using positioning in this way will make their job of descending and being born much easier.

Crowning

YOU MAY HAVE heard tell of a little thing called crowning, also known as "the ring of fire."

I will not lie to you. This is not a walk in the park. There's nothing to compare it to. The skin and muscles surrounding your vagina are stretching to allow a baby to come out. It's hard to sugar coat that to someone in your position—someone anticipating the unknown. I will though, because it is awful in the truest sense of the word.

Awful:
inspiring awe

filled with awe: as deeply respectful or reverential

extremely disagreeable or objectionable <*awful* food>

exceedingly great—used as an intensive <an *awful*ly beautiful baby>

Crowning is awful.

So, when faced with a situation which could easily be perceived as awful in the "extremely disagreeable" sense or in the "exceedingly great" sense, I'm sure by now you can guess which path I will choose. With a nod of acknowledgement to the disagreeable, I'm going the other way. Crowning is going to happen no matter how you look at it, so we might as well focus on it being exceedingly great. The way you do that is by being informed; being surprised by the intensity of crowning does not help, I guarantee it.

Remember that even though it is a moment of intensity, it is still just that: a moment. It will take me far longer to describe it than it will take for you to experience it. It's wise to make sure you have a woman that you can look in the eye at this time, one who has been where you are and lives to tell the tale! Whenever possible, a calm, supportive partner that can be your rock, should be holding your hand. Take the chance, if you can, to reach down and touch your baby's head, see if there is hair, begin bonding, this is an extraordinary experience that you are having together. Have a mirror available so your focus can be at least partly on the anticipation of seeing your baby for the first time. Listen to the excitement in the voices of the people around you, already beginning to celebrate! Push through the intensity and know that this is all normal; you will be absolutely fine.

This tissue is made to stretch—has been doing so for thousands of years—and it will be over sooner if you just welcome the intensity and push through it. Listen to the instructions being given to you. You may be asked to pant or blow, or give little pushes as the head begins to emerge, which can help to avoid tearing. You may be asked to change positions if the baby is trying to clear the pubic bone. The crowning of the head takes some time, little by little, the baby moves down, the tissue stretches and between contractions the head will sort of slide back up, giving your body time to prepare to stretch more next time, and so on.

Centimeter by centimeter, the baby's head will emerge. The head is the hardest part, once the head is out the rest of the baby usually slides out in the next push or two. You cannot imagine the degree of joy, relief, excitement, love, relief, happiness, connectedness, relief, more love, enchantment, and more relief that is inherent in this moment. It is magical.

To add to the magic, one of the most beautiful elements of this moment can be having your birth partner help to "catch." Not all practitioners are open to the practice. I recently had an experience where I asked the doctor if the dad could help catch, and she was extremely opposed. Upon further discussion, I discovered that she literally thought that I meant for her to leave the room or stand back and let the Dad wing it! It was so funny, but I clung to my composure and then asked if the dad could just participate by ceremonially touching the baby and perhaps helping to bring baby up to Mom's abdomen. She was totally ok with that, which is all we wanted anyway! It can be a powerful rite of passage. There is no real reason (other than a concern regarding the baby's heart rate or other known medical complications) why the hands of family shouldn't be allowed to instinctively reach in.

The procedure offers no benefit in routine deliveries.

Episiotomies

THIS PROCEDURE IS sometimes used to speed second stage labor, though I've rarely see it used in recent years as studies have demonstrated that the harm caused is only warranted in the case of an urgent/emergent situation. As the baby begins to show at the vaginal opening, a cut is made in the posterior of the vagina. Like all procedures, there are reasons to perform this surgical incision. All of the reasons should relate to the Mom and baby's vital signs. There is a normal amount of stress caused by the baby moving through the birth canal. The pressure on the head causes the heart rate to decelerate.

In rare cases, an old school doctor may tell you that an episiotomy speeds second stage, directs a tear toward the rectum instead of toward the clitoris, or makes suturing easier. All those things may be true, but let's elevate our expectations. First of all, our bodies are designed to stretch to allow the baby to come out. Let's just assume that nature may know a thing or two. This isn't a race; we want the tissue to stretch slowly to avoid tearing.

The threat of tearing can be used to scare you into agreeing to an incision, which is, of course, simply a controlled tear, which usually results in a larger tear than would happen naturally, that the doctor gets to bill for.

Many studies have found that the procedure offers no benefit in routine deliveries, and there is no evidence to suggest that it improves a woman's sexual function. It has also been found that women who have an episiotomy have more intercourse-related pain after pregnancy and take longer to resume having sex after childbirth.

If an episiotomy cut is made, there is more of a chance that it will become a larger tear or even extend into the muscles around the rectum. This can lead to later problems with controlling gas and sometimes stool. When no episiotomy is made and a woman is just allowed to tear, these problems are less likely to happen.

—New York Times Health Guide
http://health.nytimes.com/health/guides/surgery/episiotomy/overview.html

Tearing is a big, scary word, when we are talking about one of the most sensitive part of our bodies, especially. Let's de-mystify it. If an episiotomy is not performed and a woman is coached well at the point of crowning to slow her pushing to a pant or blow, the effects on the vaginal opening commonly range from: no tear at all, perhaps a "skidmark" or abrasion inside the vagina which does not require sutures, up to a slight tear in the first or second degree, maybe requiring a few little stitches that will heal faster because your tear will happen in the weakest/thinnest tissue.

By contrast, if I take a piece of fabric or paper and perform an episiotomy on it, then apply pressure, what will happen? You bet your ass: a big tear (3rd or 4th degree) without breaking a sweat. An episiotomy might make your second stage shorter, but you will pay for it later by having to sit on an inflatable donut for a week and experience other discomforts walking, going up and down stairs, using the bathroom etc. It is easier for the doctor, giving them a route of entry for a vacuum extractor (which is the most common reason for performing this incision whether or not they tell you about it) and a straight line for sutures. You don't really care if you have a straight line or not. The doctor is paid enough to stitch your jagged little tear. Their convenience isn't your concern.

Barring medical necessity, it's fair to expect patience from our providers and placing the patient's comfort, during the birth as well as post-partum, ahead of the schedule, provider convenience, or other incentives to perform this incision.

This irreplaceable moment should be revered and respected.

Summary

THERE ARE SEVERAL variations and a few other positions that your birth team may encourage you to try if the pushing stage is taking longer than average. Average being 2-4 hours for first time Moms. Remember that you get long rest periods between contractions here, sometimes up to 4 or 5 minutes. Generally, the pushing stage gets shorter with subsequent births.

There is no reason to have any more contractions than are absolutely necessary, so, like first stage, my advice is to use every contraction to make as much progress as possible. Use positions allowing the baby and your uterus to do some of the work. With a strong urge, use breath-holding techniques and good position to push. Relax the muscles that your baby is trying to pass through, making sure to avoid any time pressures and emotional stress. These are the surest ways to shorten second stage and get to the magic. This irreplaceable moment should be revered and respected. Through the ecstasy of being done, the bewilderment of what your body just did, the satisfaction of reaching the summit, even sometimes a certain degree of shock, you will meet your child for the first time.

What could be more important or worthwhile than that?

Homework for Lesson 6

See Classroom Resources on www.ExpectingKindness.com for
  Reading assignments
  Articles/additional resources
  Links to video's
  Exercise assignments
  Journaling prompts
  Tools for partners
  Relaxation techniques

Lesson 7

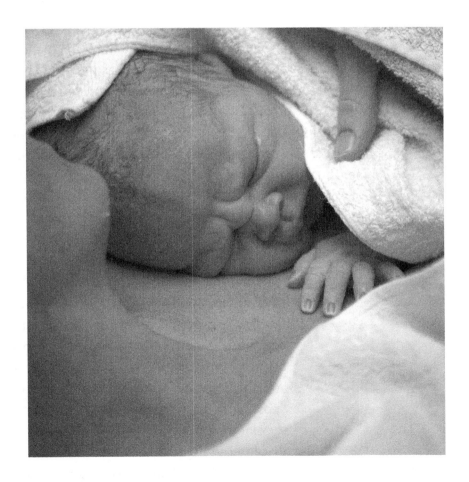

"Utter and complete LOVE... and, "FINALLY." It was like finally meeting someone that I needed to know and have in my life."

—Alesia Regan-Hughes, Mother, Artist, Reiki practitioner
on meeting her child for the first time.

Third Stage

THIS IS THE stage immediately following the birth and includes the immediate care of Mom and Baby as well as the birth (so to speak) of the placenta. There is a lot going on around you during this time as well as a lot of emotional and mental changes going on inside all of you. Of course, Mom and baby are still undergoing physical changes as well, so we will walk through everything one step at a time. There are some decisions you need to make regarding your wishes for immediate care so that you are free to focus on the first moments of your new life together instead of having to be giving constant directives to your staff.

I'm going to be bluntly honest with you now and just come out and tell you that other than the pushing of the epidural/pito-

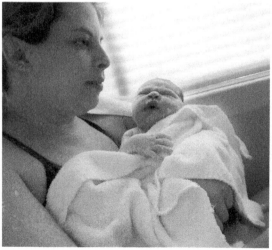

cin/episiotomy/Cesarean cycle that happens at the hospital, this period of time is the biggest challenge with hospital care under normal birth/normal newborn circumstances. I tell you this for one reason; you can instigate change. You need a very specific "post birth newborn care" plan that (barring necessary intervention) may become the standard of family centered care. You can be a part of a healthcare "kindustrial" revolution, reversing the harmful effects that the industrial revolution had on giving birth and improving compassionate care in mainstream medicine, sincerely expecting kindness.

The moments after birth

IMMEDIATELY FOLLOWING THE birth your medical team is checking the baby for the immediate APGAR scores. This score is established twice, at one minute and five minutes to check the baby's vital signs. Heart rate, respiratory effort, muscle tone, reflex irritability and color are all evaluated on a scale of 0-2, for a maximum of 10 points.

If the baby is taken away urgently following a low APGAR score, you can usually identify the urgency in the room. A real concern is evident; obviously, we want your care providers to intervene if the baby isn't responding well. Your care team is also watching and evaluating Mom for a couple specific things: bleeding, shock, consciousness level/responsiveness, mostly through observation and verbal communication. These evaluations are often completely invisible to you, because a) They happen really fast, and b) Your baby has enchanted you.

As long as everything looks healthy and normal, your baby should be able to be brought immediately up to your abdomen. At this point, your care provider will likely (attempt to) put a hat on the baby. This has become the standard of care, protocol, although the research indicates that skin-to-skin contact and a blanket over both Mom and baby in a reasonably warm environment is adequate and the hat serves no actual purpose. For bonding, skin-to-skin contact is critical and allows babies to use their senses to find milk, regulate their body temperature, heart rate and respiration. The baby is brought to the abdomen, ideally, not the chest, due to the umbilical cord still being intact. There is a very important reason to let the cord remain intact until it stops pulsing. It is providing Oxygen to your baby while he or she figures out how to breath, which can take a minute (feels like longer) to begin, and sometimes a little longer than that to work out the kinks. Some kiddos come out talking and wailing right away, but sometimes we need to encourage the baby to begin breathing by massaging and encouraging him/her. We love it when the baby starts to make a little noise because what follows a yell or a cry, is a big gulp of air. What I most often see is a baby with good color, eyes open and interacting, reactive muscle tone, good heart rate, but not breathing right away. Cut the kid some slack, leave the cord intact; newborn babies have never breathed air before.

This moment is one of the many reasons why I advocate as much as possible for drug-free births, meaning drug-free babies. The drugs used to medicate women in labor pass through the placenta and enter the baby's bloodstream. It has similar numbing effects on baby, but isn't placed locally so the effect is a more systemic general lethargy.

Effect of an epidural

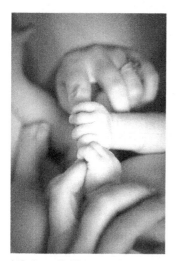

Life Actually Photography

THE FOLLOWING IS an excerpt from http://www.american-pregnancy.org/labornbirth/epidural.html:

How can an epidural affect my baby? As previously stated, research on the effects of epidurals on newborns is somewhat ambiguous, and many factors can affect the health of a newborn. How much of an effect these medications will have is difficult to predetermine and can vary based on dosage, the length of labor, and the characteristics of each individual baby. Since dosages and medications can vary, concrete information from research is currently unavailable. One possible side effect of an epidural with some babies is a struggle with "latching on" in breastfeeding. Another is that while in-utero, a baby might also become lethargic and have trouble getting into position for delivery. These medications have also been known to cause respiratory depression and decreased fetal heart rate in newborns. Though the medication might not harm these babies, they might experience some subtle effects like those mentioned above.

Might not harm? *Really?* Subtle? Last time I checked, not being able to breathe well didn't fall into the "subtle effects" category. I wonder how many women would choose epidural/spinal anesthesia if the dialogue was thorough.

Woman: I want an epidural!

OB: Really?

Woman: Yes, I don't think I can do this!

OB: There is no medical need for drugs at this time.

Woman: I can't do this!

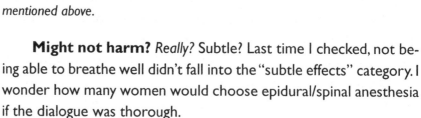

OB: It could make it difficult for your baby to breathe or nurse, but it might not harm her.

For many women, that could easily be the end of the conversation.

In the medical profession, not providing unbiased, true information that could significantly affect the decisions we make in regard to our healthcare is unethical. The emphasis on being politically correct and not making people feel uncomfortable or judged for asking for anesthesia when there is no medical indication has somehow overshadowed the fact that there are medical risks to mom and baby. When considering any intervention, the benefits of the procedure or drug should outweigh the risks to mom and baby. Even if it is just delaying it as long as you possibly can, less it always better. Turn over every other stone first, and know you are stronger than you could ever realize. It takes BIG physical experiences to realize how deep that well is.

> Leave the cord intact until it stops pulsing. Newborns have never breathed before.

The umbilical cord

WHENEVER POSSIBLE, NEWBORNS, medicated or not, should have access to their scuba tank—leaving the cord intact until it stops pulsing—until they surface and are breathing independently. Some encouragement is common, rubbing the heel to elicit a little cry, stroking the head, perhaps blowing some oxygen into baby's face, talking to the baby, but a slight delay in breathing isn't typically a cause for panic, especially when the cord allowed to pulse.

There is only one valid reasons to cut the cord immediately: **Immediate medical care for Mom or baby.** Otherwise, there is no rush and it is beneficial to allow the baby to have all of his or her cord blood/oxygen while learning how to breath. Cutting the cord immediately outside of absolute medical necessity is simply impatience on the part of the practitioner. Though most of the cord blood is transferred to the baby in the first 1-3 minutes, the cord can commonly take anywhere from 5-10 minutes to

One Tree Photography

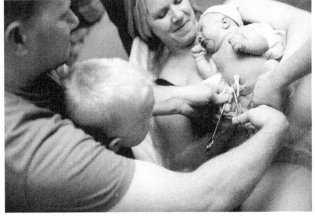

stop pulsing. In a water birth, I have witnessed a cord pulsing for a good bit longer. Even if you are collecting cord blood for storage or donation, it is unnecessary to cut the cord, as your provider can draw the blood directly out of the cord as is pulses. Much like I don't have to have my arm severed when I donate blood. I often see providers who say that is has stopped pulsing so they can save time, when I can plainly see that it hasn't. They assume that we won't know the difference. I have seen a doctor say, literally immediately following the birth, that the cord had stopped pulsing.

To prevent this from happening, ask to feel the cord (or have your birth partner do it) to verify that it has stopped. You don't have to do it in a rude way; you can ask in a sentimental way. "I want to feel it when it's pulsing and when it has stopped, I want to experience everything, I'm so curious!"

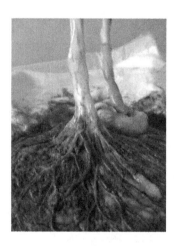

Once the cord has stopped pulsing, it is lovely and symbolic when a member of your birth team is given the opportunity to cut it. It is much more meaningful when performed by a family member or friend. I have even had the chance to cut one serving in the Doula role when no family members wanted the honor. The cord is clamped with a surgical clamp a few inches from the baby, and again with a small plastic clamp or tie, near the baby's navel and then the cord is cut between the two. It usually takes a couple snips to get through it, like cutting through a small, rubbery, rope. If we wait for the cord to stop pulsing, there should be very little to no blood when it's cut. Now baby can be brought up to the breast for a much closer look, eye contact, breastfeeding, playing, and exploring. Babies born without exposure to hours of painkilling drugs are often alert, expressive, and ready to interact right from birth.

After the cord has been cut, the placenta will soon release its grip on the uterus and be expelled. As the release of the placenta is happening, you may feel some cramping; which is a mild contraction of the uterus. This process can also take a little time, although with a new little person to focus on, it often goes by quickly. It is not safe to pull or tug on the cord to expedite the process. Some care providers do hold onto the clamp attached to the cord to provide a little tension, to see if it has released rather than trying to get it to release. For your safety (avoiding unnecessary blood loss) it's important that the placenta come out in one piece. Once the placenta releases, the expulsion is relatively uneventful. It is a soft, flexible organ, about the size of a salad plate, with no bones and is usually pure relief when it comes out. You may be asked to give a little push, sit upright or just cough to encourage it to come out.

When the placenta is out, the site where it was attached becomes a big, raw vascular open wound. Your birth team will monitor your blood flow and make sure that your uterus does its job of tightening/contracting (using massage and/or medication when necessary) to minimize the size of the uterus, and consequently the size wound inside your uterus. Imagine a balloon blown up to the size of a small watermelon, and a circle drawn on it the size of a salad plate. That's the size of the placental site before the uterus tightens, now imagine letting enough air out, so that the balloon is the size of a large grapefruit, what would happen to the circle? That's what we are going for, a much smaller wound. The massage isn't too bad, but I wouldn't call it comfortable. Even though you have a brand new, and pretty impressive pain tolerance scale, it feels weird and pretty mean to have someone poking around your soft, empty, tender belly.

> "There is no word or way to describe something so wonderful as meeting your child for the first time. I just remember being flooded with a sense of love that was so much greater than I ever knew possible." - HM

Baby's first hours

FOLLOWING THE IMMEDIATE post-birth checklist, verifying vitals, etc., is generally the beginning of the chasm between the holistic care model and the industrialized medical care model, though I've been happy to see that chasm appear to get smaller in recent years. Recent studies are now proving what holistic birth workers have believed for centuries and medical practices are beginning to move closer to more family centered care, since it's now backed by science.

Once mom and baby's wellbeing has been established, nothing else has to happen right now. The baby is at your breast, and there is absolutely no reason that he or she needs to be anywhere else for hours. The first two or three hours following the birth and the immediate care of mom and baby are absolutely priceless. Your baby, especially if unmedicated or minimally exposed, is likely to be alert, engaged, and interacting with you. I recently asked a random

"Absolutely the purest joy I've ever felt. I have never in my life felt that happy. The relief is there, but secondary to the pride I felt for US and our first biggest accomplishment as a family." - JJ

sample of moms to try to describe their feelings in that first moment. Here are the responses:

"It's different each time but for C (firstborn) Magic. Wonder. Awe. Peace." For J, my words are Frustration, Relief, Shock, Respect, Victory. (also, Big-I couldn't think of anything else except how big he was-that's included in the shock. Haha.) - CG

"Cloud 9" - TC

"Complete." - LJ

"Blessed. Miraculous. Fulfilled. Complete." - JJ

"Humbled." - SM

"Awestruck, frightened (one of the twins inhaled amniotic fluid) filled with tenderness and love." - JS

"Proud. Awestruck. Happy and sad all at once. Getting to hold E, but saying goodbye to the hiccups in my belly." - TM

"Relief. Glad both my babies were ok. Xoxo" - CA

"Overwhelmed." - CF

"Completely perfect creation" - SA

I was in awe of my daughter. I couldn't take my eyes off of her. Totally in love. - KD

"Earth-shaking. Awe, like seeing someone you've known and loved your entire life for the first time! My first thought both times was, "I know you!!"" - EC

"Pride, love, spiritual, thankful and amazement! For the first born I felt that a real family was born between E and I. This was overwhelming LOVE!" - MS

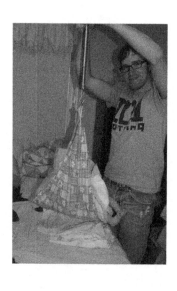

Creating the space and time for your new family to be fully immersed these first moments, and give the creation of a new family the reverence it deserves, should be at the top of everyone's priority list. I can't think of anything more important. All the things on the lists of things to do and boxes to be checked can wait for a while.

You have discoveries to make—critically important things like, looking into your baby's eyes, truly the window to the soul. You must count the toes and discover the utter miracle of little jagged fingernails, peek under the hat to see every little hair on his/her head, touching and caressing and kissing the softest sweetest cheeks on the face of the planet, looking to see if your baby has the family dimples, comparing the: ears, chin, toes, eyes, lips to your own. Making sure that the sex of the baby was what you thought it would be, or discovering the sex of the baby for the first time. Watching the baby see you for the first time and realizing the immediate familiarity, sensing how he or she reacts to your voice, your touch, and your kiss. Looking at your partner and feeling the powerful connection inherent in having gone through this together.

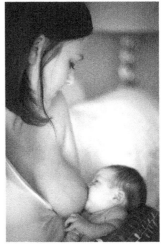

Life Actually Photography

These are not small things, although not often prioritized or valued in the sense of planning ahead to make sure you have the time to honor them. Even acknowledging that there are situations where Mom is tired, recovering, needing an emotional respite before engaging into the Mommy role, having this time allows you to let the bonding happen as it comes, organically, without any externally forced delays, nor any pressure to bond quickly. Calm, relaxed, and restful, take your time.

As a doula, I see part of my job description as being an event planner. Do you want a picture at this moment? Do you want special music playing? Do you want certain people present? Do you want to have the sex announced by someone special or discover it yourself? Do you want to announce the name? Have cake, a toast, a prayer or a welcome ceremony for the birth celebration? This is a moment you will re-live and re-count a thousand times or more in your lifetime, more than any other event in your life. Create a beautiful memory by stating a clear expectation.

The lists of things that will eventually have to be done are somewhat dependent on your chosen birthplace, but the list may include the following:

- **Breastfeeding**. Although many women feel strongly about immediate breastfeeding, there is usually no huge urgency. Once the umbilical cord is cut, the baby nuzzling and sucking on the breast stimulates oxytocin production and can help the uterus stay firm. You can certainly encourage the baby to latch on at any time. It is natural for a newborn to seek out the breast and given the opportunity, may even work their way to the nipple independently. Let the baby determine the urgency, he or she may just want to look at you for a while and that's ok too.

- **PKU.** This is a heel prick to test the baby's blood for Phenyl-ketonuria among other things. Testing for PKU is the standard of care. It involves a heel prick and blotting a little blood onto a strip for testing. There are long-term risks of undiagnosed PKU, some examples are: mental retardation, ADHD and other behavioral disorders, seizures, and eczema. While the test is a reasonable precaution it does not need to be done in the first few minutes, hours, and sometimes, days of life. The rate of false positives in the first twenty-four hours is higher, so there is often a follow up test in the first week anyway and there is no immediate risk to your baby.

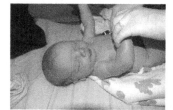

- **Eye Prophylaxis.** This antibiotic ointment is put into the baby's eyes to protect the baby from blindness caused by exposure to gonorrhea and/or chlamydia during the birth process. The ointment blurs the baby's vision for about ten to twenty minutes. Once the initial bonding period has passed, and you are all ready for a nice restful nap is a perfect time to administer this treatment, if you so choose.

- **Vitamin K.** This is commonly a poke, an injection in the baby's thigh. The intent is to thicken the blood to prevent internal bleeding caused by birth trauma or HDN (Hemorrhagic Disease of the Newborn). Again, the decision is yours to make, but there is no immediate risk if there is no immediate concern for the well-being of your baby. You should be advised if there has been a potential trauma (like vacuum/forceps) that would increase the risk of an internal hemorrhage. Otherwise, should you choose to do it, the injection can be delayed for a few hours and done while baby is nursing, and if you do a little finger compression at the site just before the injection and immediately after, sometimes they don't even notice. There are options for oral administration, both for baby at the time of birth, as well as for Mom in the weeks leading up to delivery. Talk to your care team and weigh all the risks and benefits, as the rate of absorption in the baby is lower with the oral options.

- **Hepatitis B vaccine.** If Hepatitis B is detected in a prenatal blood test, meaning a pregnant woman is Hepatitis B positive, an early vaccination (usually within twelve hours) is critical, the vaccine in any other case is purely precautionary since Hepatitis B is transmitted through sex or shared needles. If you have reason to believe that your baby may be in close contact with people engaged in "risky behaviors" you may consider this vaccine, but aside from maternal infection, there is no immediate risk and it can be delayed/refused if you wish.

- **Newborn Exam.** Many hospitals lead us to believe that the baby will be examined while still in our arms. This is sort of true and untrue. The APGAR test, done in the first few moments of birth is sort of an exam, and is generally done with baby on the abdomen, that is the "true" part. When I'm talking about the newborn exam, I mean the head to toe once over that is done on the bed next to mom at home or birth center births, but for some reason, in hospitals, baby is taken to an exam table (often across the room) with bright lights and warming lights. It's fine, I guess, and family is usually invited to stand next to the table and touch the baby, but mommy is often excluded because it tends to be done in an efficiency model; check out the baby while mom is getting her stiches, or going to the bathroom, or waiting for the placenta, or taking a shower. In a family-centered model, moms and dads get a guided tour of baby's body. You gain confidence in caring for your newborn.

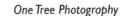

One Tree Photography

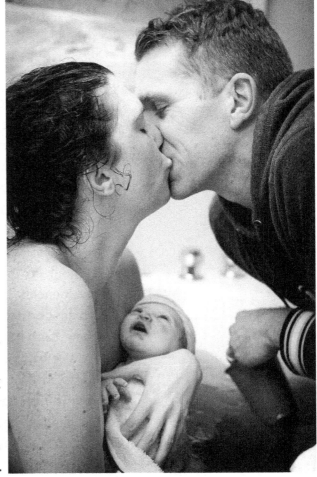

Seeing what is normal, knowing what they are checking for helps inform new parents and may also bring up questions that new parents wouldn't otherwise think of. I advise making sure that you are present for this!

- **Bathing.** Generally, at a home birth or birth center birth, the only "bath" your baby may be given is the one that he is born into, but in many/most hospitals, the bath is a standard of care. I think this is odd for a variety of reasons. First and foremost, it is a robbery of the very first "first." It is one of the first of the things we take pictures of—moments that help build our confidence in our partners and ourselves. Why do we let total strangers bathe our babies? They don't touch, talk to or hold them the way you will. Some of the best memories of parenting are born out of not knowing what the hell you are doing and figuring it out together. Second, the hospital is kept pretty cool, and in an environment where there seems to be hyper attentiveness to any deviation from the narrow spectrum of "normal," getting the baby wet in a cool room (increasing the risk of a drop in core body temperature) seems like a very strange practice, specifically unadvisable in the first six hours of life. Third, the baby isn't dirty. There may be a little birth gunk in baby's hair, there may be a little vernix (a coating on the baby's skin protecting it from the water environment), which is beneficial if left alone or rubbed into the baby's skin like lotion. There is also the concept of the microbiome, beneficial bacteria passed from mother to baby as they pass through the birth canal, studies are showing that it is best to wait at least 24 hours to bathe your newborn to give them all the possible benefits. There is nothing going on that a loving caress by mommy or daddy with a warm washcloth in a warm room at home can't handle, in the first few days of life. Avoiding submersive baths will also help the cord stump to dry out and fall off faster, YES to that!
- **Swaddling.** Some babies do find comfort in being swaddled, but initially, the baby benefits from skin to skin contact; the radiant heat from mom's body (or even dad's bare chest in the event that mom is receiving care and can't do it yet) helps the

baby to regulate her body temperature, heart rate and respiration. If there is a concern about baby not being warm enough, add a warm blanket over both baby and parent.

- **Gestational Diabetes testing.** This test is generally only suggested if you have a baby with a very low birth weight or a very high birth weight or if Mom has been diagnosed with Diabetes or Gestational Diabetes, as all can be indicators of potential diabetes in the newborn. The risks to the baby if undiagnosed are significant, so when requested, this is a test with an actual degree of urgency, it isn't necessarily an emergency, but a reasonable precaution. Feel free to try to delay it, your staff will tell you if they believe it to be more urgent than you realize.

- **Circumcision.** I know this is hot topic, it always sparks controversy. This will be an editorial piece, do with it what you will. The most important things I want to tell you in consideration of this procedure follow:

  ¤ STUDY. Consider it and weigh the factual pro's and con's the way you would consider any other *aesthetic* surgery on a newborn.

  ¤ It is painful for him. At least as painful as it would be for any other male, he has all the same nerves as anyone else; he is a complete human being, just smaller. He may be more sensitive, because of the fresh sensitivity to the outside environment; even a diaper must feel like sandpaper to a newborn compared to the soft, smooth, maternal environment.

  ¤ It opposes the Medical Code of Ethics to remove healthy tissue.

  ¤ Know this: It is not your penis, it's his. This is a very big decision you are making on his behalf. It is your responsibility to educate yourself about both sides. You may have to answer his questions later, especially if he disagrees with your choice. However, invested you may be personally, no matter how much pressure from friends or family you may be under, it is not your body.

  ¤ "Looking like Dad" is a baseless argument. Why are people so fixated on this? How often do you compare penises with your Dad? Ew. By the time he is old enough for his penis to remotely resemble an adult male penis, it is totally inappropriate to be comparing, in fact, I would argue that any comparison at any time is inappropriate. Seeing differences is healthy, comparing/competing is wrong. I would also like to say here that I have met MANY women who have opted out of this decision with the rationale that "the dad has a penis, so he should make the decision." You are the mother! You spent a considerable amount of time during this pregnancy building the foreskin, which is unlikely an accident of nature, it is meant to be there. You are often the one who will be: changing the majority of diapers, re-dressing the wound, listening to (and feeling) him cry in pain, comforting him, potty-training him, taking him to his pediatric visits, teaching him about his toddler/childhood erections, and eventually, sex. You get a solid vote. If you are divided, perhaps your son should get to be the tie-breaker, at least. It can always be done, but it can't easily be undone.

¤ Infection risk. A ridiculously slight increase in the rate of a *treatable* UTI does not rationalize cutting off a part of your son's penis, which will then be exposed to fecal matter in a perfect bacterial breeding ground. Bathe your baby/child regularly, have regular medical exams and be aware of signs of UTI. Consider that your child may also acquire an ear infection, eye infection, any infection from a cut or scrape. We don't perform an amputation of any other body part due to a potential infection.

¤ Teasing in school. The national rate of circumcision has dropped significantly so make sure you do your homework and find out if your child will be in the minority by being circumcised, as indicated by current data. The other consideration is this; your kid might get teased in school. If it's not his penis, it will be his shirt, or his glasses, or his hair color, or his grades, or the way he walks, dances, jumps, catches, likes musical theater, his intellect, bad haircut, etc. Kids can be cruel; it's not a reason to amputate part of your child's penis. It's a reason to teach your child about compassion and kindness.

Your care provider has the best interest of the baby in mind.

¤ There are risks in circumcision. There is even a mortality rate directly associated with circumcision: shock, blood loss, anesthesia, and infection being the "cause of death." It is admittedly a very small risk, but people circumcise every day out of fear of other small risks, so it is as notable. There are also significant risks from botched procedures, which can lead to painful urination, painful erection, painful sex if untreated, or a slew of other risk factors to face in surgical reconstruction with anesthesia.

¤ Regarding circumcision, there are considerations for risk of exposure to disease, medical conditions, geographical location, hygienic conditions, and cultural/religious expectations. Please just don't use old, outdated, geographically insignificant, baseless, emotional, one-sided information to support a personal bias in making this aesthetic decision on behalf of your son.

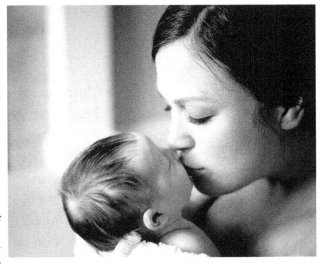

Life Actually Photography

Even religious circumcision has some gray area as I've been told by religious practitioners. A marking, for example, doesn't necessarily demand the full removal of the glans. I'd encourage research and consulting with your faiths specific guidelines.

Hopefully, it isn't an overwhelming list of things to make decisions about. It will take a little time and discussion with your partner and, perhaps, your midwife or doctor, but the time it takes to make decisions now you will get back later. Knowing how you feel about these procedures ahead of time will prevent the time being taken away from your first hours, days and weeks with your baby, to have it all explained to you and trying to make decisions in a somewhat dreamy, other-worldly state of reality.

There are some circumstances in which being opposed to certain newborn procedures will require you to sign forms and potentially be subjected to lectures from staff. Knowing specifically why you are opposed, having the forms signed ahead of time, and presenting them confidently will help to avoid some unnecessary dialogue. Some families opt to waive some/all of these procedures and do them with their family doctor or pediatrician. Having a doctor (medical or naturopathic… or both) already hired for follow up care is another tool that you can come prepared with. In my experience, the hospital staff is more comfortable entrusting the baby into your care if they know you have taken that first step.

It is important to remember that your care provider has the best interest of the baby in mind, don't take it personally; they see a lot of hard situations that create the need for caution. Have compassion for their experiences and come prepared to demonstrate that you have made thoughtful, informed decisions; proving that you, too, have the best interest of your baby in mind even if your opinion of what that means differs from theirs.

Homework for Lesson 7

See Classroom Resources on www.ExpectingKindness.com for
    Reading assignments
    Articles/additional resources
    Links to video's
    Exercise assignments
    Journaling prompts
    Tools for partners
    Relaxation techniques

Lesson 8

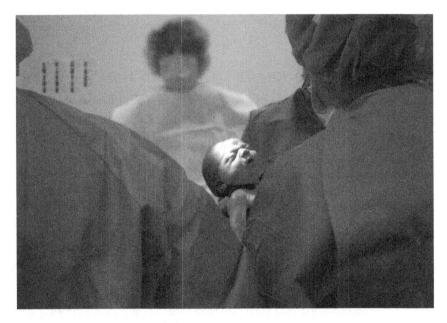

"We should constantly be asking ourselves 'Is this an improvement, or are we making things worse?'"

—*The Business of Being Born*

Variables in Childbirth & Active Management of Interventions

As we mentioned in the introduction to the first lesson, there are no guarantees. You can follow every guideline, exercise every day, eat 100% organic foods, have the best prenatal care, take the best class, read everything you can get your hands on, and occasionally things come up anyway. You can't control everything and that's an important lesson to carry into your parenting career. The best you can do is advocate for yourself, know what you want, know why you want it, and try hard to get it. But always keep an open mind. Complications are possible. Your task is to make sure you aren't being manipulated into interventions that aren't medically indicated, especially those that may increase the risk of other interventions. Make sure you have turned over every stone, trying the least invasive intervention first and only by necessity, escalating. It can be hard to let go of an ideal, but when the health and safety of mom or baby requires it, the decision is simple. Cautious compliance is the name of the game. Some interventions characterized as "standard of care" or "hospital policy" are applied universally to women in labor prior to any diagnosis or medical necessity because of the need for consistency in a hospital, but many of these practices can be negotiated.

A couple examples:

1. I.V.: An I.V. may be a "required" preventative intervention. The reason given is to prevent dehydration or to have it in place in case of an emergency. An I.V. may not seem

You are pregnant—not sick.

108

like that big of a deal, but it limits your mobility, making it harder to change positions for contractions. It's natural to feel like the doctor is an authority but you're pregnant, not sick. Drink plenty (16oz/hour) of water and stay active so hopefully there is no need for an I.V. to keep you hydrated. If you are tethered to a pole with a IV in your hand, moving around, changing positions to cope with contractions, getting in and out of the tub/shower, and even using the bathroom becomes a production. The perception of being a confined patient, combined with other commonly used tools like a continuous fetal monitor and a blood pressure monitor, easily leads to the sense of being tethered, confined, and helpless, as opposed to empowered and instinctive. There are degrees of compliance here. If you are trying to avoid confrontation at check-in, or if there is an indication that you *may* require fluids or antibiotics, opt for a compromise. A Heparin Lock gives the Doctor or Midwife a connection for an I.V. if it becomes necessary without having to be hooked up to the fluids, lines and poles all the time. Another compromise might be agreeing to fluids, but not continuously. The fact that they put an IV in doesn't mean you have to receive bag after bag until you give birth.

2. Induction or Augmentation: Oxytocin is a naturally occurring hormone, sometimes referred to as the "love hormone." It is produced to bond with your baby, stimulate milk production, and help with contractions. *Synthetic* oxytocin, marketed as Pitocin is often used frivolously to "manage a labor." Using this drug, doctors can sometimes make contractions (although not necessarily labor) begin or make it stronger/faster. Pitocin is unpredictable and does not create the smooth, wave-like contractions of natural labor. It creates a constant seesaw trying to balance the levels with what you are naturally producing. Once introduced through an I.V. you are required to have continuous fetal monitoring… because there are risks to the baby which require constant evaluation… which also limits your

mobility. Combined with the unnatural contractions, this series of events frequently creates the perceived need for an epidural.

3. There are, of course, medical reasons to use Pitocin, but scheduling your labor is not one of them. If its use were limited to actual medical necessity, the rate of epidural anesthesia and Cesarean section would decrease significantly. There are so many less invasive options that could be applied prior to pitocin, Some include: Waiting till labor kicks in on its own, encouraging contractions (ideally in the morning so we're not losing sleep over bouts of contractions that may or may not become labor) using tools like acupressure, acupuncture, chiropractics, a Foley bulb catheter (a little balloon that when inserted into the cervix and inflated), brisk walks, sex, suppositories to soften/ripen cervix, can all help to induce/encourage labor. That's quite a few stones to turn over before you submit to pitocin.

VERY IMPORTANT

Know what "normal" means to your doctor or midwife. Before labor, ask, "What is the range of normal?"

Giving full informed consent.

WHEN YOU USE this language, you state powerful intention of being an active participant in your care. Your Mantra:

"I am informed, I am not a typical compliant, patient. I am not placing blind faith in medical expertise and giving up all responsibility so that if something goes wrong I can blame it on the doctor or hospital later. I want to collaborate and take on reasonable responsibility for the decisions made on behalf of my child and myself. I have hired my provider to assess the safety of my labor and birth and I want their professional opinion. I will ask questions, I will challenge them. I will allow non-emergency intervention only if they can convince me that it is in my best interest or the best interest of my baby. I trust them in an emergency situation to take excellent care of us."

You never have to say any of this to anyone; it is implied when you tell your care provider that you want to be given the opportunity to give full informed consent if a complication arises that may require an intervention, when it is safe to do so.

Excerpts from the American Medical Association

Informed Consent

Informed consent is more than simply getting a patient to sign a written consent form. It is a process of communication between a patient and physician that results in the patient's authorization or agreement to undergo a specific medical intervention.

In the communications process, you, as the physician providing or performing the treatment and/or procedure (not a delegated representative), should disclose and discuss with your patient:

- *The patient's diagnosis, if known;*
- *The nature and purpose of a proposed treatment or procedure;*
- *The risks and benefits of a proposed treatment or procedure;*
- *Alternatives (regardless of their cost or the extent to which the treatment options are covered by health insurance);*
- *The risks and benefits of the alternative treatment or procedure; and*
- *The risks and benefits of not receiving or undergoing a treatment or procedure.*

In turn, your patient should have an opportunity to ask questions to elicit a better understanding of the treatment or procedure, so that he or she can make an informed decision to proceed or to refuse a particular course of medical intervention.

This communications process, or a variation thereof, is both an ethical obligation and a legal requirement spelled out in statutes and case law in all 50 states. (For more information about ethical obligations, see the AMA's Code of Medical Ethics, contained in the AMA PolicyFinder. Providing the patient relevant information has long been a physician's ethical obligation, but the legal concept of informed consent itself is recent.

—The American Medical Association's Council on Ethical and Judicial Affairs
http://www.ama-assn.org/ama/pub/physician-resources/legal-topics/
patient-physician-relationship-topics/informed-consent.page

Principles of Medical Ethics

1. *A physician shall be dedicated to providing competent medical care, with compassion and respect for human dignity and rights.*
2. *A physician shall uphold the standards of professionalism, be honest in all professional interactions, and strive to report physicans deficient in character or competence, or engaging in fraud or deception, to appropriate entities.*
3. *A physician shall respect the law and also recognize a responsibility to seek changes in those requirements which are contrary to the best interests of a patient.*

4. *A physician shall respect the rights of patients, colleagues, and other health professionals, and shall safeguard patient confidences and privacy within the constraints of the law.*

5. *A physician shall continue to study, apply, and advance scientific knowledge, maintain a commitment to medical education, make relevant information available to patients, colleagues, and the public, obtain consultation, and use the talents of other health professionals when indicated.*

6. *A physician shall, in the provision of appropriate patient care, except in emergencies, be free to choose whom to serve, with whom to associate, and the environment in which to provide medical care.*

7. *A physician shall recognize a responsibility to participate in activities contributing to the improvement of the community and the betterment of public health.*

8. *A physician shall, while caring for a patient, regard responsibility to the patient as paramount.*

9. *A physician shall support access to medical care for all people.*

> *—"Code of Medical Ethics." American Medical Association, Council on Ethical and Judicial Affairs, publication ES21:01-396:60M:10/01.*
>
> *For more information on the Code of Medical Ethics, please visit http://www.ama-assn.org/ama/pub/physician-resources/medical-ethics/code-medical-ethics/principles-medical-ethics.page*

These two excerpts demonstrate the actual standard of care, as directed by the AMA, and confirm that you have actual rights to expect and receive respect and medical care, even while valuing a holistic, family-centered philosophy. Unfortunately, in many cases, in order to get the care you are entitled to, it is critical that you know both your rights and your providers' ethical and legal obligations to their patients. Family centered, holistic medical care should never be an oxymoron.

Self-advocacy

NOW YOU HAVE a basic understanding about the care Doctors and Midwives should be providing, without you having to ask for it. How do you use this information to advocate for yourself in a situation where a variable may require you to accept a deviation from your birth plan? How do you stay in the driver's seat and prevent straying from your course any more than is absolutely necessary?

The following list is a compilation of my own, based on decades of service as a doula and details many of the more common variables in childbirth that can come up as well as typical procedures to be aware of so you can protect yourself against the frivolous "standard of care," "policy," or "procedural" use during the course of your labor.

Important: There are occasionally emergencies as well as non-emergency reasons to intervene in childbirth. Being cautiously compliant is necessary because:

1. Many Cesarean Sections are actually caused by unnecessary early intervention. All treatments have potential risks and potential benefits. There is no guarantee either way.

2. If you avoid unnecessary interventions (to the best of your abilities) and an emergency happens which requires an intervention, you can accept the deviation openly, knowing that it wasn't caused by elective interventions. No regrets.

3. True emergencies aren't subtle. Whether caused by other procedures/treatments or not, you can easily recognize when a true complication is upon you. Your care providers appear serious; they may be conferring with other doctors or midwives; they are unwilling or too busy to answer your questions or discuss alternatives; they are moving faster; more staff may have entered the room, and there is a palpable sense of urgency. These scenarios are rare in healthy uncomplicated pregnancies.

Common Variables, Complications and Procedures

Post Date:

You have passed your EDD (estimated due date) as determined by date of conception (if known), ultrasound, sonogram, or measurement of fundal height. The medical community has held fast to the arbitrary number set by Dr. Franz Karl Naegele, a German obstetrician, in his 1830 book for midwives as 280 days from the onset of the last menstrual period (LMP). Many professionals hold this date in near-religious reverence. But full-term has long been considered 38-42 weeks and at best, the 40-week target could be considered "average." On the other hand, a 1990 study reported by the American College of Obstetricians and Gynecologists showed that the median gestation for white, first-time mothers in America was actually 288 days or 41 weeks and a day. While the study focused on a single race, there is no evidence that the term varies based on race. The chart shows the *average* delivery date at 40 weeks, but you should count on 41 being more likely.

There are concerns on both sides of the spectrum as we move further out to the edges, on the earlier side, we must be aware of the potential for: low birth weight, higher incidence of jaundice, small mouths (making latching a little more challenging), less endurance for feeding/wakefulness, and lack of lung maturity. On the other end of the spectrum, we must watch for: larger babies, calcifications on the placenta, decreased amniotic fluid, fetal distress. In this scenario, 40-41 weeks is ideal and the further away you travel from it in either direction, the more risks there are.

Options:

Plan to go past your due date (it's typically based on the 40-week textbook model). If diagnosed as Post-Date, ask:

- "Could my due date be wrong?"
- "Does my fundal height match the ultrasound estimated due date?
- "As long as my baby and I are healthy, what is your policy regarding going past my EDD?"

Fear of having a big baby is often fanned at this time. Using Ultrasound to establish the baby's size is wildly inaccurate. Its margin of error (especially close to term) is very high, in the range of 3 pounds (1.5 pounds on either side of the estimate). That is a margin in the range of 25%! I can give you that kind of accuracy just looking at you. I recently heard a birth story in which the mother elected for a Cesarean based on the baby's estimated size of 11 pounds, the baby weighed 7.5 pounds at birth. This is not a rare outcome because in medical care they often diagnose the worst-case scenario and then back up as new data presents itself.

Remember, first time mom's often go one or two weeks past due date

Begin to explore natural methods of encouraging labor; old wives' tales have sometimes been passed down for good reasons! After you've tried your mother-in-law's banana bread, spicy Thai food, and a car trip over bumpy roads, talk to your care provider about the possible benefits of: nipple stimulation, sex, acupressure massage, pedicure, herbs, acupuncture, brisk walking, sex, sex, sex.

Premature Rupture of Membrane (PROM)

A premature rupture of membranes, or PROM, means your bag of water leaks or ruptures—SPLOOSH!—prior to the onset of labor. *Options:*

Make sure you are consulting with your birth team and stay at home as long as they will let you. (Fewer germs there.) Some possible options are:

- Try staying off your feet for a while (in the case of a small rupture/slow leak).
- Avoid baths (shower is ok) until labor has begun, stabilized, and your care provider gives you the green light.
- You can try some techniques to try to encourage labor prior to pressure for induction. A few things you might try are: Nipple stimulation, acupressure, herbs (under advisement from your provider), acupuncture, pedicure. Not intercourse, this time. If you are trying to do anything to get labor going, I advise doing it in the morning after a "good" night of rest. Once you get things going, we don't know how long you will be working, so try to begin while you are well-rested. You may be required to have I.V. antibiotics approximately every 4 hours if you tested positive for Strep B, but this doesn't necessarily require you to check into your facility. 4 hours is a long time.
- While at home, watch your temperature and continue to drink water, contact your birth team and go if they have specific concerns, although you may choose to just go into the office or into triage, rather than checking in for the long haul.

Artificial Rupture of Membranes (AROM)

Rupturing the membranes with the "crochet hook" is often done as a means of augmenting labor. It's effectively a "wild card." It has some very specific applications that may be beneficial, but carries risks of placing you on a clock, as most facilities have a limit as to how long a woman can labor with membranes ruptured, other risks include: cord prolapse, and baby being forced down into the pelvis in a potentially more challenging position. If suggested, ask questions about the risk vs. reward for both doing the procedure, as well as not doing it. Then make an informed choice.

Options

You may simply politely decline this one in most cases. If there is continued pressure to "do something" to get labor moving faster, try responding with sincere patience and the willingness to allow your labor to follow its natural course. Press back against "statistics" with your individuality. "I am not a textbook." You can further stall this procedure by offering a number of other preferred methods you wish to try first to augment labor: walking, nipple stimulation, foot and ankle massage, shower, squatting, standing, swaying, etc. The bag, if left intact provides some cushion from the intensity of the contraction and also usually encourages nice, even pressure which is ideal for uniform dilation. It will almost always break on its own. Having a baby born in the bag, or with part of the bag still presenting ahead of the baby (also called born in caul) is not common, but it is also not a complication. There are actually some very interesting beliefs surrounding being born with a caul, also called a veil. Some believe it is a gift that brings psychic abilities, seeing auras, having predictive dreams, leadership qualities, among others. It is very rare, but certainly nothing to fear. There are circumstances in which we choose this intervention to avoid other more invasive tools, like pitocin.

Herpes

Herpes sores in the vaginal area may be life-threatening if transmitted to the baby. Do everything you can do to avoid an outbreak in the weeks leading up to your EDD. Active sores present at the time of birth are a strong case for a cesarean section.

Herpes simplex type 2 lesions (sores) may be life-threatening to the baby.

Options:

- Take medication to treat outbreaks.
- Minimize stress to reduce the likelihood of outbreaks.
- Keep up on current research regarding new tools and techniques that may protect baby from exposure during a vaginal delivery.
- Prepare for the increased probability of Cesarean section delivery and plan for other ways to maintain the important issues on your birth plan.

Occiput Posterior (OP)

When the baby is head down, but facing the abdomen instead of the spine. Occiput Anterior is "spine facing" and ideal.

Options:

- Prevention: If the baby is in a posterior presentation, talk to your birth team about things you can do, like pelvic tilts for example, to encourage baby into a better position for delivery. Doing pelvic tilts can get the baby up and out of the pelvic basin and encourage baby to sort of drop into the hammock of the abdomen. Find ways to hang out comfortably in positions that apply gravity in the right direction: abdomen toward the ground. Use pillows, massage pads, whatever you can to create space for the belly while in a face down position… without lying *on* the baby. There is also a technique called Rebozo that involves a strip of fabric and using a rocking motion to get baby up and out of the pelvis to help him realign. If you are diagnosed with an OP baby, find someone who has specific training. Many midwives and doulas have been trained in this gentle, non-invasive technique. During labor, babies move a spiraling action throughout their descent, so the fact that he/she may be OP at some point, does not necessarily mean that will be the case throughout labor and birth.

If your baby has a very strong opinion about staying in this position:

- Due to the increased intensity of contractions, additional support in the form of family, friend or hired Doula is recommended.

- Mom will probably require more physical support in the form of direct backpressure near the sacrum and/or pressure against the hip bones, pushing in and pulling back. Putting mom into the hands and knees position can take some pressure off the back and gives her support team easy access for the pressure. Laboring in water (even if you don't plan to give birth there) can also be very helpful.

Breech

Any presentation in which the baby is "upside down". There are a few versions of breech. If baby is booty first or foot/feet first he is considered a breech presentation.

Options:

If you know about this position in advance, there are a lot of things to try to get the baby to turn. Of course, talk to your care provider prior to trying anything. Some examples:

- Handstands in a swimming pool, ice on the top of your tummy while submerged belly button deep in a tub of warm water, your partner can talk to the baby near the pubic bone, music low on your abdomen, acupressure, acupuncture, aromatherapy, hypnotherapy, chiropractic care.
- Finally, as a last resort, an external version in which an Obstetrician, when safe, physically moves the baby by external deliberate pressure while sonogram and external monitor assess baby's wellbeing and tolerance of the procedure.
- If baby is still breech at term, most are delivered via C-section. Vaginal breech is *possible* if all the planets align and you have an uncommonly knowledgeable, experienced, skilled, and willing midwife, OB, or perinatologist.

Rapid Dilation

If mom appears to be moving through the signs and symptoms of labor rapidly it may be more intense with long contractions that are close together. It is often an emotional challenge because of the ambiguity of the length of first stage labor, she may assume that it will be this intense for the average length of first stage and become discouraged with her inability to handle these intense contractions for a supposed long period of time.

Options:

- Keep up with consistent verbal and physical support and keep her morale and confidence strong. In this case you will usually find yourself at your birthplace and with more support earlier because she will demand it, so you won't be handling a baby coming out at the speed of light by yourself.

- Be ready to catch. It's not impossible that you could find yourself catching a baby. That is always a possibility when you are attending a woman in labor. There are several sites on the web that you can visit, or ask your Doctor or Midwife for a specific set of emergency childbirth instructions to follow and keep it handy. It's mostly a list of things to NOT do, and if the baby is really coming, you should be on the line with your care provider and/or a 911 emergency dispatcher for guidance while you wait for skilled support to arrive. Precipitous birth aside, rapid dilation has its own set of challenges, not worse, or better, just unique. You'll simply jump to the skills and tools for active first stage labor and transition sooner in the process. It's a good idea to re-read the stages of labor chapters as your due date approaches so the information is fresh in your mind.

Slower Labor

A labor that is considerably longer than average, average being 24 hours from start to finish. This diagnosis depends heavily on when we start counting! It is very common to start the "labor clock" at the first sign of any sensation that differs from the common Braxton hicks. My recommendation is to ignore "maybe" signs, and wait until your contractions do not slow, stop or change in response to your position or change in activity, and are consistently following that 5-1-1 rule discussed in "First Stage Labor". Anything leading up to that point could still be part of the normal/healthy process of preparing for labor and may come and go. Get as much rest or sleep between contractions either way, whether it will or won't become labor will make itself known in time. Set yourself up to have the energy for the long game, if needed, and know that even naps in intervals add up, and even a collected hour or two of sleep can carry you farther that you think. A well-rested, well hydrated, well-nourished woman is less like to have a long drawn out early phase of first stage because her body is energized and ready to go. A marathon runner who doesn't sleep the night before is unlikely to be performing optimally on race-day. If you happen to be the privileged few, who prepare for the marathon, and have to run it, you still have some things to consider.

Options:

A slower early phase may be identified by a lack of increase in contraction frequency, intensity and duration. Make sure her labor isn't slow to progress because of external reasons: her position, her ability to relax, any stress caused by her surroundings. Watch her reaction to her contractions, is she pulling up or fighting the contraction? If all of the external factors are fine and there are no medical complications, you can continue to use strong support. This may be a reason for communicating with any helpers you may have lined up to provide back up support. Talk in between contractions about relaxing her whole pelvic floor in response to the contraction: drop the shoulders, relax the jaw, sink down and open up for the baby.

Encourage her to conserve energy by resting or even sleeping between contractions and re-energize her if she seems to be fatiguing with some electrolyte enhanced fluids. My favorite energy tools are: Coconut Water, Honey dissolved in warm water, Vitamin Water, Recharge (sport drink) which you may need to dilute by about half for a laboring woman to cut the sweetness. Give her fluids and sugars, like a hummingbird. It is critical that she stays hydrated. Additionally, sustained energy provided by a protein source can also become important; yogurt (I prefer Greek yogurt for extra protein), peanut butter toast, or other nutritious, easily digested foods can be very sustaining.

Occasionally, a slow labor is a true complication and there is a reason the labor isn't progressing, or the baby isn't descending. A nuchal cord, cervical abnormality, pelvic structure, and baby's presentation are a few reasons. C-sections are sometimes recommended simply out of impatience, so make sure you have your informed consent questions ready.

Labor Respite

Occasionally contractions will begin, and continue for a long enough period of time that it can appear to be actual labor. When contractions start and stop, it is healthier to accept the contractions for what they are: bouts of contractions that may cause some dilation, but have not yet progressed into the type of ongoing labor pattern that is necessary to produce significant change in the dilation of the cervix. All contractions are beneficial, so if they come, welcome them, and if they go… Take the break!

Options:

You can use many of the techniques used to begin labor, although, when a break in the action happens, I would advise you to consider it a gift. Many (almost all) women wish for a break during their labors. TAKE A NAP! As long as there are no complications, just rest and be thankful. After your nap, you can try non-invasive techniques to encourage labor again, or just act as if you had a nice dress rehearsal and welcome your labor whenever baby is ready.

Failure to Progress

Means failure to dilate fast enough, usually comparing you to a textbook or a statistic. Of course, this can only be diagnosed if you are letting your provider check you. There is a lot of power in limiting your cervical exams. If you are checked and dilation is unchanged remember that overall progress may be achieved in other areas: like baby's position, effacement, texture (softening or ripening) of the cervix, cervix moving forward (if posterior). Failure to progress is often given as a reason for a Cesarean surgery or Pitocin augmentation.

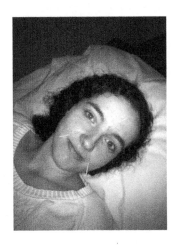

This is the single most common reason given for intervention in labor. I have personally witnessed many beautifully managed labors that ended in lovely vaginal births lasting well over the prescribed average. The first thing on my list in this situation is figuring out if Mom is feeling safe, and if not, what can be done to increase her sense of security and comfort. Don't get psyched out by the clock, and don't allow yourself to be bullied into intervention because the staff is bored, remember you can go back home! For intervention,

wait for a medical diagnosis that does not rely on statistical/potential outcomes or theoretical implications or intuition.
Options:

The options here are the same as for slow labor, as slow labor is often the basis for this official and demeaning diagnosis.

Assessing Pain Tolerance

Unless you are using Pitocin, in which case an increased level of pain is common, labor with above average levels of pain, or pain that is not wavelike, rising and falling intensity may be an indication of a complication. Normal labor does not typically involve sharp pain.

Make sure your care provider is checking baby and mom's vital signs at the prescribed intervals. If all signs are good, continue with strong support and position and activity changes that may make mom more comfortable. Shower or bath may be the most effective. Remember, barring a complication, contractions are generally most effective when they are very strong, so intensity is what we are going for.

No one is in your body but you. You alone must assess your pain level and your pain tolerance. Having said that, the pain scale commonly applied in labor is flawed. A 0-10 scale is only accurate if you have been in extreme pain, and many of us haven't been. There are certainly circumstances in which women may need to use some pain management. I only suggest that we begin to try tools and techniques first which do not fall into the category of controlled substances. If you throw every tool, technique, activity, and position you have at your pain and nothing helps, you may be better able to accept the risks and liabilities inherent in choosing pain relief.
Options:

Prior to epidural anesthesia, spinal anesthesia or morphine

- Sterile water injections: An intracutaneous injection of sterile water near the sacrum which alleviates back pain in labor for up to two hours and can be repeated as necessary.
- TENS: A pad placed in 2-4 locations around the sacrum that deliver an electric pulse which increases the production of serotonin and activates the opioid receptors creating a mild analgesic effect without using controlled substances.

- Acupuncture (if provided)
- Massage: See transition massage sequence, sometimes this kind of physical and emotional touch/support is required throughout much of active labor.
- Freedom of movement: taking walks outside, around hallways, in circles around your kitchen island at home. Change of scenery, combined with various movements, swaying, stair climbing, hula circles, yoga ball sitting and leaning. etc. It often feels better to be active.
- Eating/drinking lightly to maintain endurance
- Bath/Shower: Shower as much as your hot water tank will allow, save the tub for "the natural epidural", when you feel like you can't do it anymore, it will provide significant relief when saved for those moments.
- Nitrous Oxide: Not used widely in the US, yet, but becoming more and more common. I want you to be a part of normalizing this tool because it is far safer than the dangerous controlled substances currently used to manage normal labor discomforts in the U.S. It is also *very* temporary, leaving your system in just a few breaths, allowing you to self-regulate and use the pain relief just at the exact moment you need it, ideally through the peak of the most intense transition contractions and/or at crowning.

Meconium in the Amniotic Fluid

Most often it's normal, but may rarely indicate distress. When the bag of water breaks, if there is any particulate matter or if it appears to be brown or green in color, it is a good idea to communicate that to your birth team. They may wish to listen to the baby's heartbeat more regularly. If they do not appear concerned, you can assume it falls into the category of normal. The possible risks are that the release of the bowel movement can itself be an indicator that the baby is stressed, which would be confirmed by monitoring the baby's heartrate. Additionally, there is some concern that at the time of birth, the baby may aspirate (breathe in) some fecal matter which can (rarely) increase risks associated with blockage of the airway and infection.

Options:

- If there is meconium, allow your birth team to listen to baby to verify his or her wellbeing. It will allow them to have confidence, assuming everything is healthy, and to make informed decisions that are in the best interest of the baby if he or she is not tolerating labor well.

- Knowing also enables your team to be prepared and have the supplies necessary at the time of birth to respond quickly to baby's needs if necessary.

- Talk to your providers about what the range of normal is in regard to the baby's heart rate throughout the stages of labor and the descent through the birth canal. Knowing what is "normal" will help you (or your partner) evaluate if there is a real need to intervene on the baby's behalf, or if we should be using our informed consent tools.

- A true urgency/emergency isn't subtle, so if there is an absence of that sense, feel free to question intervention. If you feel that sense of urgency, you can trust that there is a risk that warrants action.

Baby Can't Fit Through the Pelvis

CPD (cephalopelvic disproportion) is often diagnosed and given as a cause for a Cesarean surgery. In the area where I work, I commonly see this issue being diagnosed very prematurely, sometimes as early as 6-7 months gestation. It isn't even always given as a diagnosis, but rather a seed of doubt, planted early, and then fertilized and watered throughout the pregnancy. My opinion is this is usually pure speculation using tools that have a wide margin for error. Furthermore, it is often "diagnosed" prior to the cartilage softening, prior to the hips shifting, and prior to squatting while pushing. It ignores the individuality of each woman and fails to acknowledge the increased weight of the baby opening the hips further or the use of upright positions and movement to allow the baby to wiggle down in there. Except in rare cases such as childhood malnutrition, or unmanaged/advanced Gestational Diabetes, true CPD is highly unlikely and can really only be assessed after a generous amount of time in true second stage labor. Some doctors abuse this diagnosis to schedule their cesareans without having to wait through hours of labor. Obstetricians may not value natural vaginal birth above their own personal and professional schedules or management of perceived or potential liabilities.

Options:

If you have a care provider that is scaring you about the size of your baby, (remember that 7.5-9.5 pounds is normal) or the outlet of your pelvis, get a second opinion. Don't accept your care provider undermining your confidence based on speculations. Do not get your second opinion from your OB's colleagues as they are unlikely to contradict him or her. Go somewhere else. Do not engage in dialogue about your ultrasound with a technician, they are not qualified to interpret or use the data to diagnose and often cause unnecessary worry with casual commentary on what things "could mean". See a midwife. See a perinatologist. Even if there may be a differential between the pelvic outlet and baby's size, the labor process still has value in preparing your baby to breathe air and stimulates changes in the body for life outside the uterus. Even if it ultimately ends in a cesarean, you will have given your baby a healthy "head's up." As long as Mom's and Baby's vital signs are good, there is no harm in pushing and giving your body a chance. Assessing a baby's size with late term ultrasound is often inaccurate. The margin of error is 1.5-2.0 lb on either side, so baby could be 9 lbs., or it could be 7.5. Needless cesareans are scheduled and performed frequently to treat this commonly inaccurate diagnosis. I hate to see women scared away from labor on the off chance that her baby may be larger, and then ushered into the operating room only to find that her baby was significantly smaller than estimated.

Fetal Distress

Fetal distress refers to an unborn baby not tolerating some aspect of labor: the contractions, the head compression when descending into the birth canal, a compression of the cord in descent. It is diagnosed by a fetal monitor; either intermittent fetal monitoring with a fetal stethoscope (although not often used during labor), doptone (handheld) ultrasound monitor, or by use of the continuous fetal monitor (the one with the belts). There is controversy in

What is considered to be normal variation in fetal heart rate during active labor?

the use of continuous fetal monitoring because there are normal variations in fetal heart rate and constant scrutiny is likely to result in noticing some variation outside the range of "normal," even if it is still healthy.

Options:

First of all, this is an important discussion to have with your care provider beforehand. What is considered to be a normal variation in fetal heart rate during active labor? What is considered normal during transition? What is a normal variation during pushing? Know what they may be looking for and, if a blip on the radar happens, be aware of the things that you have control over. Position and breathing are the most important and effective tools in your belt. Make sure you know what the circumstances are that would require your care provider to intervene.

If there is time for discussion, for asking questions, there may be an option to change position, use oxygen, or massage baby's head (even inside). As much as possible, try the non-invasive techniques first. If you are being instructed that it is indeed an emergency, obviously do whatever they tell you to do. Again, a healthy baby is our first objective.

Ultrasounds. Ultrasound can be a valuable diagnostic tool; however, the FDA has repeatedly refused to approve the use of ultrasound on women during pregnancy. Its frivolous use coupled with a broad range of inexperience analyzing the data, and a significant margin of error means parents need to be very discerning throughout pregnancy and labor when ultrasound is suggested. Even experienced practitioners acknowledge a significant margin of error in ultrasound diagnosis for everything from fetal weight, to due date, to the sex of the baby. There is a potential bias toward intervention and the data is sometimes used to support a pre-existing agenda.

Doptone Monitor. This hand held fetal heart rate monitor is most often used for intermittent monitoring of the baby. It can be used to listen for more prolonged periods of time if there appears to be some kind of concern. Doctors, midwives, and nurses may choose to listen to the heart rate between contractions and continue to listen through a contraction to listen for good variability. They want to see that the baby is active and that he or she reacts to the pressure of a contraction, within the normal range of course.

A fetal heart rate (FHR) during labor ranging from the 130s to the 140s with some variability is considered ideal. With changes in pressure (bag of water rupturing, baby moving into the birth canal, stronger contractions or changes in contraction from first stage to second stage) we expect to see some changes in the FHR, but it should recover to close to normal as the baby recovers from the change in environment. If the old fashioned, non-ultrasound, fetal stethoscope is not an option, intermittent use of the Doptone monitor is my next choice.

External Fetal Monitor. In high risk situations, the constant monitoring of your baby using ultrasound can at times allow women who might otherwise be advised to have a surgical birth, to labor and give birth vaginally. It allows the doctors to scrutinize the baby's well-being and intervene if indicated, saving babies who might not otherwise survive. Unfortunately, the technology is universally applied to most women in labor, and the continuous scrutiny of a healthy baby often causes the "worst case scenario" mentality to intervene in a situation where the variation in the fetal heartbeat could be normal, even if it isn't "textbook." The medical community acknowledges that this scrutiny increases the rate of unnecessary C-sections. In low-risk situations using intermittent fetal monitoring using either the doptone or the external fetal monitor to periodically check on the wellbeing of the baby is certainly wise, but when determining whether continuous fetal monitoring is advised the questions to ask are:

- Could it be normal?
- Is my baby in distress?
- Is this routine?
- What, specifically, is the concern?

One tool in my belt is this: Decline the use of continuous fetal monitoring, but give your staff permission to listen to the baby's heart rate at any interval they feel is necessary using the doptone monitor or the sensor from the external fetal monitor, minus the belt. You have just declined being strapped to a belt and connected to a machine, while still empowering your team to use their best judgment; they just have to stand there and do it rather than rely on technology. What this actually accomplishes is eliminating the convenience factor. Your team will not stand there and hold the monitor on you for twenty minutes, forty minutes or continuously if it isn't absolutely necessary. It also creates an opportunity to ask questions to a captive audience. You (or your insurance, or some combination) will pay somewhere in the ballpark of $7500-$10,000 (without surgery) for the birth experience. DO NOT be bullied into believing that they can't afford to provide attentive care.

Internal Fetal Monitor. This tool is an electrode, a small coil that is screwed into the baby's scalp. Again, this is a tool that has very specific applications. This is a reasonable risk to take if your team cannot find the baby's heartbeat and are determining whether or not to move to an emergency cesarean. Sometimes the baby's heart rate is hard to find, especially once he or she has dropped down into the birth canal and the pelvic bones obscure the ultrasound signal. There are varying degrees of skill in all levels of your care team. New or student midwives, less experienced nursing staff, even newer obstetricians have been known to be unable to find a steady heartbeat. Make sure you have an experienced medical professional verifying necessity and performing these risky procedures.

Vacuum Assisted Delivery or "Operative Vaginal Birth." This is a tool that I want you to avoid if at all possible. Its use should be limited to: A. Baby is crowning and at the perineum in distress; or B. You have tried every imaginable position to get the baby past the pubic bone and you are faced with either the GENTLE application of this tool or cesarean. I can't think of any other reasons to use it. The determining factor is the following question: Does the risk of the use of this tool/intervention outweigh the risk of not using it. This thing is traumatic to the baby experientially, if not medically. A suction cup is attached to the top of the baby's head and then the doctor pulls.

Please consider the following: There will usually be an episiotomy (to get the tool in there) and a high likelihood of a 3ʳᵈ or 4ᵗʰ degree tear because of the unnatural speed bringing the baby out coupled with the pre-started surgical tear. It can have an effect on the baby as well in the form of spinal subluxations (which can lead to pain and a very fussy baby later), it can also cause cephalo-

It is NORMAL for a first time mom to push for an average of one to three hours.

hematoma as well as intraventricular hemorrhage. These risks are increased when the internal fetal monitor has been "installed". This tool is sometimes applied due to simple impatience. It is NORMAL for a woman, especially a first-time mom to push for an average of one to four hours. That is normal and don't let anyone tell you otherwise. If there is distress in the baby, or the mother, those are reasons to intervene in the safest possible way, but again, impatience based solely on statistical evidence, personal experience, or pure impatience are not good enough reasons to take these risks. Please respectfully ask to be given adequate information so that you may give full informed consent. Again, if there is time to ask questions, that tells you about the degree of urgency.

Forceps. The risks for this procedure as well as the protocol to follow prior to agreeing to its application are similar to the vacuum because the intervention would be performed for the same reasons. It's just a different tool—an "old school" version of the vacuum/suction tool. Be informed enough to offer full informed consent.

If it is determined that the use of one of these tools is medically indicated, allow your care provider to use the tool with which he or she has the most experience and the most confidence in.

VBAC. Vaginal birth after cesarean. As stated in the foreword, I am not going to rewrite the book on certain subjects. There are amazing resources out there written by experts in this particular area of obstetrics. If you have found a care provider that will support your pursuit/trial of a VBAC, and your pregnancy has been uncomplicated, there is no reason to plan your birth any differently than any other natural childbirth. Just be forewarned that there is a significantly higher incidence of cesarean section when you have already had one. The risk of a uterine rupture is slightly higher, but not always a reason to give in to the pressure. It can be hard to tell if a doctor is really, truly, concerned for your well-being, or just finds it easier to schedule your delivery at his or her convenience. Apply all the informed consent skills you have learned. Question. Make them convince you that a repeat cesarean is safer by comparing the risk to benefit ratio of both VBAC and Major Abdominal Surgery and make an informed choice.

Cesarean Section. The big one, the one we all really want to avoid, and with good reason. This is the primary reason to limit the other interventions that increase the risk of distress, slow progress, and exhaustion that are often at the root of surgical births. This is major abdominal surgery, although it's treated somewhat like an outpatient procedure in many cases. After the surgery when the post-operative care is being discussed, or when you get home and require constant care and pain relief, or when you can't comfortably hold or carry your baby, you realize that you are, in fact, recovering from major surgery. Attempting to prevent this intervention is the reason many women choose to try and train for a natural birth.

A surgical birth should always be the last resort. It should be performed out of true medical necessity only. One of my biggest obstetric peeves is when a cesarean is proposed as a preventive course of action. Preventing what? A cesarean. "I'm concerned that if I continue to let you push like this, you may become too exhausted and ultimately be unable to deliver vaginally." This is a real conversation; I've seen it. I call this person a surgical predator—preying on your fear that after hours of pushing, you might have a cesarean anyway.

By avoiding many of the previously discussed interventions and limiting the amount of medication, unnatural contractions, and stress induced by both Pitocin and the epidural, we are less likely to face this one. No guarantees though, and when a cesarean becomes truly necessary, not speculatively or potentially necessary, and we have applied our skills to be certain that it is in the best interest of Mom and/or baby, we do have to be prepared to change gears.

All interventions, including cesarean section, have their place, and when necessary we are free to be deeply grateful for the science that made it possible, the anesthesia, the art of surgery, the sterile environment, and of course the steady hands, quiet confidence, and gifted precision of your operating room staff.

If you are afraid of a C-section, I urge you to let that go! None of our efforts to avoid a C-section are about fear. It's all about risk management. In an uncomplicated labor and birth, adding unnecessary interventions simply adds risk. When the risk of the intervention is lower than the risk of not performing it, we do whatever is safest for Mom and baby. That's it and that's all. A cesarean section is not something to fear, but something to avoid if the risk to benefit ratio supports it, which is true most of the time. My only wish is to be a part of a movement that limits this surgery to when it is absolutely necessary. We want to minimize the risk and potential long-term effects for mom and baby and eliminate the frivolous application of surgery used to defer the pain of labor. Recovery from this surgery is a factor to consider, especially when you include the fact that you have to also care for a newborn as you recover. A new mother doesn't get the luxury of real recovery time. It takes six to eight weeks is to recover from abdominal surgery, but there is no "time off" in motherhood. Baby requires around the clock care. If you are considering a cesarean as a means of avoiding the pain of labor, or interrupting the ongoing discomfort during labor, think again. You may be in pain for weeks after surgery. It's not a fair trade.

If we have arrived at a medical need to perform this type of birth, it's time to embrace it. If you have written a birth plan there are probably still MANY elements of the plan that you can maintain, although dim/candle light isn't among them. You can kindly request that because of all the changes in your plan, that your staff honor and respect the few items on a short list of things that will enable you to celebrate the moment. The list may include:

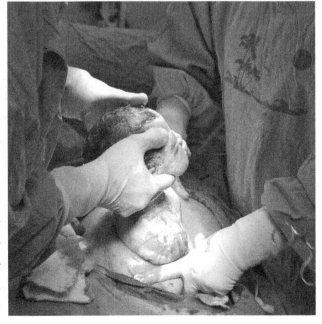

- Dad/Partner present. You may need to sign a medical durable power of attorney to assure their admittance into the OR, though not often necessary unless they are using general anesthesia. The common reason given in that scenario is that Mom will be sleeping and doesn't need coaching. Mom is not the only person to consider. I would argue that it is kinder to allow someone to witness the birth so that the story can be told. Every birth has inherent beauty and the story is important. Additionally, as long as baby is healthy, he or she should be placed immediately on Mama's chest (which will require some assistance), or in the arms of their other parent, sitting close to Mom's head.

- Doula/additional support present. If the baby needs to be taken for evaluation, one person should go with the baby and one stay with Mom. The doula may be asked to wait outside the OR, in full gear, ready to enter and stay with Mom if her primary person had to go with baby. Some ORs are smaller than others. In my experience, the decision of who and how many are allowed in is generally made by the anesthesiologist. Of course, the attracting bees with honey analogy is ideal, and certainly we should be commanding this in the kindest possible way. However, when necessary, I have had some success insinuating that it feels discriminatory to allow a woman who has no complications and is having a vaginal birth to have her doula with her, but to take that vital support, built over hours and hours of time spent laboring together, away from a woman who needs the additional support the most, more now than ever. It's almost a pleading if it comes down to it.

- Taking pictures. This is still the birth of your baby, and you should be focused on celebrating that, even if things don't go according to plan. If you are squeamish, black and white photos allow you to easily focus on the baby.

- Video: Most operating rooms won't allow video of the surgery itself, but may allow video of the baby immediately following the birth. Using your phone's camera makes this a little easier to get away with.

- Managing the environment: Some women respond well to play by play of the process, a rehearsed procedure like cesarean often leads to a confident surgeon who can provide a reassuring commentary, comforting, kind, and sometimes even feeling like OR stand-up comedy, which may seem weird, but may be quite nice. It cuts through the anxiety. Other women want quiet so that they may employ rehearsed relaxation techniques, or listen to music. Please do not hesitate to ask for what you want.

- Even in a surgical birth, you may elect to let the umbilical cord pulse. Most of the baby's blood is transferred in the first 1-3 minutes, try to negotiate for as much time as possible.

- Making the announcement of either the name, or the sex, or both, should be Mom's privilege or the privilege of her birth partner. This keeps some part of the birth personal, a celebration, and a little ceremonial. You can have a Mufasa moment in the operating room or wait till you are in the recovery room together to have a private moment.

- If baby is fine, he or she can be placed across your chest on the operating table or handed directly to your support person to hold near your head while the surgeons finish up. It is common for the nursing staff to keep the baby in a warming bed nearby: doing the newborn exam, checking boxes, dotting i's, and crossing t's that can easily be done later. It is *efficient* to "take care of all of the details" while mom is being sutured. Efficiency isn't important at this moment. Mom has just made an incredible sacrifice and as long as baby demonstrates a solid APGAR, she deserves to have her baby to gaze at, kiss, nuzzle and even be given a free hand to hug her baby. Prioritize the emotional part of giving birth, especially if it has to happen in operating room.

- Hold off on non-essential newborn procedures for a couple hours when possible. After your surgery, which usually takes around 30 minutes (once begun) where you have hopefully spent 15-20, minutes looking at your baby, you will be taken back to your delivery room or to a recovery room. Take some private family time to regroup, adjust, debrief, bond, cuddle, share, nurse, and get to know your baby. You will be in the hospital for a minimum of 24 hours post-surgery, usually upwards of 48. There is no reason to hurry. Your friends and family, the lactation consultant, your coworkers, your spiritual or religious community, can come later. The nurses can poke the baby's heel later. They can check the weight, height, head circumference ALL LATER. Take your time. Make memories. No matter what the birth experience is, find all the beauty in it and celebrate that. Learn from any part of the experience you feel was not beautiful and make it purposeful.

Lesson 9

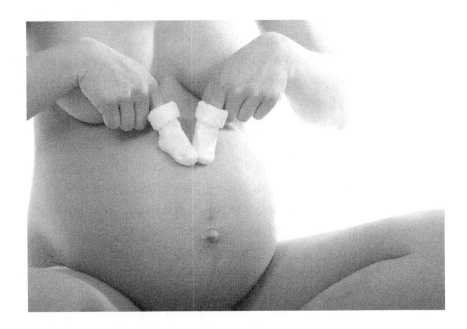

"When enough women realize that birth is a time of great opportunity to get in touch with their true power, and when they are willing to assume responsibility for this, we will reclaim the power of birth and help move technology where it belongs—in the service of birthing women, not their master."

—Christiane Northrup

Writing your Birth Plan

Write two separate birth plans.

WHAT IS A Birth Plan? The birth plan is your contract with your birth team. As a doula, I consider this plan to be my job description. All birth professionals should take them just as seriously. Discuss your birth plan with your birth team ahead of time.

The birth plan is a tool that will walk the birth team through your labor desires and give them ideas regarding comfort measures you find helpful, words and touch you like, or don't like, positions you think you will feel good about, etc. You know yourself better than anyone, and once you have a thorough knowledge of the labor and birth process, you are in a unique position to help your birth team help you. Additionally, the birth plan states your preferences regarding medical care and the immediate care of your baby.

Once in active labor and in the haze immediately following the birth, your ability to advocate for yourself and give specific feedback and instruction regarding your care will be limited. Having made decisions ahead of time and writing them down as simply and clearly as possible allows your team to know and understand your wishes without having to pester you while you are trying to let go and give birth or get to know your new little family.

Generally speaking, you should write two separate birth plans. One is for the uneventful, uncomplicated birth process, no matter where you plan to deliver. The expectation of family-centered, holistic medical care doesn't discriminate against birth locations. The second plan will provide your staff with directives if a deviation from your birth plan becomes necessary. If you are planning an out of hospital birth, this second plan is largely intended for a situation in which a transport to a hospital becomes necessary. For those planning in hospital births, it is a back-up plan in case circumstances require you to make informed choices regarding a deviation from your original plan. This secondary plan allows you to answer all of those pesky "what if" questions that you invariably have running through your mind anyway, and puts them into a framework where you can set them on a shelf and know that the answers are there if you need them.

For many years I have been challenged regarding my belief in writing a detailed Birth Plan. The popular criticism is that women with birth plans will be disappointed if there is a deviation from the plan. I find this argument to be incredibly condescending.

You are not naïve. You are not expecting everything to go exactly according to the plan. You are expecting kindness, compassion, and care, and to be a part of the decision-making process, when possible and safe. You are taking responsibility for your health. You are becoming an informed consumer and making conscious, informed choices about your wellbeing and the wellbeing of your children. You are acknowledging the medical expertise of your care providers, while still expecting to be heard, valued and respected. You want your practitioners to understand that your expertise about your own body—as well as your intuition, instincts, and opinions—when combined with a thorough understanding of the birth process can be a powerful asset.

You are taking responsibility

The birth plan changes the "assembly line" and the "doctor as authoritarian" model of care, ultimately making the experience more fulfilling for everyone involved. It's not as efficient, probably doesn't make the hospital as much money, and may take more emotional energy; but we pay a lot for our care and it is a fair expectation.

Two concise, detailed birth plans, ideally one page each.
- Birth Plan A: How could your birth be perfect?
- Birth Plan B: How do you want to be taken care of if intervention becomes necessary?

Birth Plan A

ESTABLISH THE ASSUMPTION that your child's birth could easily be uncomplicated and within the range of normal, no matter where you plan to deliver. Therefore, you will want this, this, and this. You know you may change your mind. You know the plan doesn't guarantee anything. It's a plan, and isn't carved in stone. Don't use the word "unless" in plan A. You only need to state ONE TIME that you will be flexible should a complication arise. Don't say, "I don't want Pitocin… unless my Doctor thinks it's necessary," or "I don't want pain medication unless it becomes necessary for the health of me or my baby." It's goofy that we have to say it at all.

A woman who is willing to experience a natural childbirth, believing that it is in the best interest of her baby, would also be willing to accept necessary interventions if circumstances arise that make it safer to intervene. Your goal is always the best for the baby. I've never met a woman who was willing to sacrifice her baby for a natural birth.

So, when writing this ideal birth plan, use a warm, "asking" tone with the underlying expectation that your wishes will be honored. Write Plan A as a letter to your birth team to help form a good relationship. Save the bullet-points for plan B.

Sample Birth Plan A

_____Family, Wishes for our Child's Birth

Dear _____ and staff,

My name is _____. This is my first pregnancy and I am looking forward to having your support and expertise as I labor and give birth. We don't know the sex of the baby, but call the bump _____. We have taken a comprehensive class and trained for a natural childbirth because I am terrified of needles and don't want to have a cesarean unless it is an emergency. **We will, of course, be flexible in case of an emergency; I understand that circumstances can come up that may require intervention. I would like to be given the opportunity to offer full informed consent if a complication does arise.** As long as my labor remains uncomplicated, I wish to labor with my support team and ask that you refer to and respect this birth plan.

Birth Team:

Mother:_____Partner:_____Doula/Assistant Support:_____

Primary care Doctor/Midwife_____

First Stage Labor:

We plan to labor at home as long as possible, and will be in contact with you once my contractions are five minutes apart and lasting forty-five to sixty seconds to let you know what is going on as per your request. I will also call if anything out of the ordinary happens, blood, water breaking, lack of movement etc.

We want to wait and come in to the birth center when my active labor is well established, but before transition. Your help determining the right time to check in will be deeply appreciated. I would like to have the freedom to go home if I am less than 5cm dilated.

While at the birth center I plan to use the following comfort measures:

Showers, changing positions, warm compresses, cool washcloths, massage with comfrey oil, guidance to release tension, music (iPod playlist titled "First Stage").

My labor mantra (to repeat during challenging contractions): "And the day came when the risk to remain tight in a bud was more painful than the risk it took to open" (Anias Nin).

Do not offer me medication. I empower you to challenge any requests I might make for medication in a moment of weakness.

As my labor progresses, I believe that I will want to have access to the tub, and have continuous support, talking me through the contractions and providing physical support. I usually hold tension in my lower back and in my jaw and I like firm pressure on my low back.

I am open to some alternative pain relief, like TENS or Sterile Water Injections and would consider Nitrous Oxide during transition if I really need to take the edge off. If I can labor through it in the tub, that would be best.

I want to labor with freedom of movement and without any time limits being placed on me.

Second Stage Labor:

Once I am fully dilated, I wish to wait until I have an uncontrollable urge to push and allow the baby to labor down so I can save my energy in case this stage is longer than average. I have a play list of calming music also, (Second Stage) but I'm not sure I'll want it on.

I may just want it quiet, so please ask. I will want lights dimmed and candles lit. (flameless if in hospital)

I have practiced pushing technique and I believe that I will want to have freedom to push in a variety of positions. I may prefer: Side lying, supported squat, and semi-reclined. I am very open to your suggestions for efficient positions; please make suggestions if you feel that there is a position that will be more effective.

When the baby is close to crowning, I would like to have a mirror available so I can see my baby. I would also like to have my Mom present at the time of birth, please invite her in (if she isn't there already) as soon as we can see the baby's head. PG rated pictures/video are OK.

We would love for my partner to be a part of "catching" the baby, however ceremonial, helping to bring the baby up to me as he or she is born. We want to discover the sex of the baby on our own, please do not announce it at birth. As long as we are both healthy, I would like to have my baby with me immediately and continuously. We want the cord to stop pulsing prior to being cut and we would love a chance to feel it pulsing and feel it when it's done.

In the event that baby requires care, my partner is to remain with the baby at all times.

We plan to breastfeed exclusively, no pacifiers, formula or water without informed consent.

Eye Prophylaxis can be administered at two hours, Vitamin K administered while breastfeeding

This is our first baby, we would value having the complete newborn exam done with the whole family present so we can learn about our baby from head to toe. We want to understand what is normal and what may be abnormal, and your guided tour would be invaluable. If it is necessary to have the baby in a warming bed for the exam, please move the bed so I can see, or wait until I can walk and stand.

All other non-emergency newborn procedures will be completed with our pediatrician, Dr. _____ at _____within the first week.

Sincerely, _____

Your initials here indicate that you have read and agree to help me achieve as much of this ideal birth as is healthy.   _____   _____   _____

Birth Plan B

EVEN IF THERE is a diagnosis that requires a deviation from the above plan, you don't have to give up everything. Obviously, you'll make necessary concessions for safety, but you need to define what will make this new situation a beautiful memory regardless of circumstances. Some circumstances only require a change in geography, a slight spike in blood pressure may force you to move from a home birth or birthing center to a hospital, for example, and if you can avoid unnecessary routine procedures, geography may be the only change. Sometimes we have to concede to tools to get labor going in an effort to avoid bigger interventions, for example if you have been goofing around with contractions that are not bringing cervical change, but keep you up at night for a couple days, you may benefit from something to kick the labor over and help you avoid a cesarean due to simple exhaustion. Just having a need for some augmentation doesn't necessarily mean it has to be Pitocin. Even if Pitocin is used as a last resort, it doesn't mean you have to have it on continuously once things start moving. It also doesn't require you to have an epidural. It's harder to cope but not impossible. Make sure you keep your "questions to ask in order to give full informed consent" handy so you will feel confident in your decisions. No regrets.

This secondary plan doesn't require all the thoughtful detail; you have already declared the ideal in your primary plan. If your transport or escalation of care is not an emergency, your care team will have time to read your primary plan first. If circumstances require an escalation or if there is an emergency, Plan B becomes a simple bullet list of directives regarding the medical care of you and your baby. Plan B should be considered an addendum to Plan A, not a replacement.

Sample Birth Plan B

In case a medical need arises that requires transport or other intervention(s) in my labor/delivery, I expect that whenever time allows, that I be given the opportunity to offer full informed consent for all procedures, both maternal and newborn. If I am unconscious, I empower my partner to make decisions on my behalf. Please see the attached Medical Durable Power of Attorney.

The following is a list of requests based on the potential need for an escalation of care. I realize that I may need to concede some of these, but because my birth has turned out quite differently that I had hoped for, I will be very grateful for anything you can do to help me maintain as many of these requests as possible. While you may forget about my birth by tomorrow, I will relive it and recount and retell it for the rest of my life.

This story matters to me.

> *IMPORTANT*: **We will, of course, be flexible in case of an emergency; I understand that circumstances can come up that may require intervention. I would like to be given the opportunity to offer full informed consent if a complication does arise.**

- If there is no emergency, please read my Plan A and help me maintain as many elements (even if some flexibility is required) as possible. Do this before any "routine" interventions are performed.
- I want my partner and my doula to remain with me at all times
- I would really appreciate attention to the atmosphere, dim, candlelit, and relaxing to the extent possible. I brought flameless candles just in case.
- I want to limit interventions to those that are absolutely necessary.
- I prefer a Hep Lock to continuous I.V. fluids
- You may monitor my baby at any interval you feel is necessary using the doptone or external fetal monitor sensor, but I decline the use of belts or straps and continuous fetal monitoring.
- I prefer to try all non-invasive augmentation methods before resorting to Pitocin (your suggestions will be welcomed and appreciated)
- I do not want Morphine. Please do not offer it.
- If pain management becomes necessary for prolonged pain above my tolerance level, I prefer to use a tub, TENS, Sterile Water Injections, and/or Nitrous Oxide. If that is ineffective I prefer a walking epidural, providing enough relief to give me some respite, but ideally, I still want to feel my body and my labor enough to move and push effectively. I know that you can't guarantee that, but please try.
- I want to turn over every stone before submitting to surgery.
- Even if I am medicated and don't need constant backpressure, I still want to have continuous physical and emotional support. Please don't assume that the epidural will replace that. Hand massage, stroke my hair, neck massage, things I can still feel.

- If surgery becomes necessary, I want an epidural only, no morphine.
- If time I allows, I would like a few minutes alone with my partner and my doula to talk through and accept the new plan.
- I would love to have the surgeon give me a play-by-play during surgery and would appreciate lighthearted, casual, conversation or music in the OR to give me something to focus on. I've heard that it can sometimes even be kind of "fun" in there?
- If my baby requires immediate care, my partner should accompany the baby and leave my doula to take care of me until we can all be together again.
- If the baby is healthy, I want to have my partner hold him/her skin to skin and sit by me as the surgeon closes. I would like one hand free to touch my baby.
- Please let me remove the oxygen mask so I can kiss him/her.
- I want to discover the sex of my baby on my own, please do not announce it.
- My partner and I want to announce the baby's name once we are back in the recovery room, with video rolling, so please don't ask.
- I plan to exclusively breastfeed, no bottles of formula or water without specific consent and medical necessity.
- All routine newborn procedures should be delayed at least two hours, or until consent is given.
- We request to have a private family bonding time as soon as we are all together again in the recovery room. No interruptions please.
- We plan to check out as soon as possible, please have all forms and discharge procedures signed early so when we get the "go ahead" we can just go.

Thank you so much for doing your best to provide both the best medical care and to still create an environment that allows us to have a loving welcome for our child. We will always be grateful for the care and compassion you offered us.

Sincerely,

_____

Make it your plan

PLEASE DO NOT just copy either sample above into a word processor and hit print. These are just some ideas to help you organize your wishes. State them clearly and as kindly as you can while still asserting your understanding of your rights and a clear expecta-

With your birth plan, you have truly become a medical advocate for yourself and your family.

tion of being treated with both medical expertise and with dignity, respect, and compassion.

Even when birth becomes a bit of a medical experience, it is still a human experience. It is uniquely feminine, astonishingly powerful, and beautiful. It offers those of us who are privileged to be there, the opportunity to witness real self-sacrifice and true love. To witness this, is a gift and that gift should be valued. No matter how many births a practitioner has attended—and it can range into the thousands—we must always remember that it is the only chance you will have to labor and give birth to this baby.

With your birth plan, you have truly become a medical advocate for yourself and your family. Building a thorough knowledge of your body, the range of normal in medical situations, and the common variables, will prepare you to make future medical and life decisions for your growing family, for yourself, for friends, and perhaps even for aging parents, aunts, uncles, and grandparents.

I hope you feel empowered to ask the tough questions. Take the time to surround yourself with care providers that share your philosophy of family-centered, holistic care. Their willingness to listen to you, educate and inform you, and treat you as an irreplaceable member of your own care team is vital to your well-being and will help change the status quo of the birth industry.

Homework for Lesson 8/9

See Classroom Resources on _www.ExpectingKindness.com_ for
Reading assignments
Articles/additional resources
Links to video's
Exercise assignments
Journaling prompts
Tools for partners
Relaxation techniques

Lesson 10

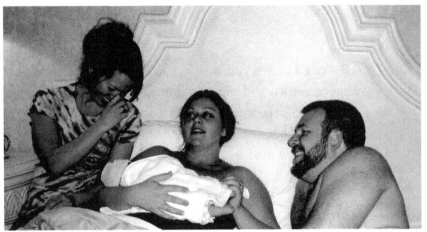

Life Actually Photography

Every Child

May every child have fresh food and clean water.

May every child have a safe home.

May every child receive a truthful education.

May every child be appreciated for being alive.

May every child have heartfelt friends and time to enjoy them in a calm place.

May every child have the chance to discover and respect the natural world found in wild places.

May every child have the chance to love, care for, and protect animals and plants.

May every child have the chance to learn the skills needed for a lifetime of harmless livelihood.

May every child know the satisfaction of living without anger.

May every child know both sides of kindness and understanding.

May every child bloom.

—Buddhist Prayer

Having your baby

BEFORE I LEAVE you with a short list of experts that I trust will enhance, enrich and simplify your early parenting, I have a little advise, parent-to-parent, that I wish to offer. These are the things that I wish I had been told—or was told and wish I had listened to—when I was a new mother.

Surviving week one

THINK SURVIVAL IN the first week. It is not always sunshine and roses; it's a big transition and the challenges can catch you off guard. You will be tired, from the pregnancy and from the birth, immediately followed by round-the-clock care of a newborn. Even if the birth is uncomplicated you should expect some challenges. Your hormones will change rapidly, making you moderately to considerably off balance. Expect it. Your body will sometimes be sore and will certainly feel weird. Doing normal things will take more attention that you expected. The pressure of nourishing and nurturing a new baby can be surprising.

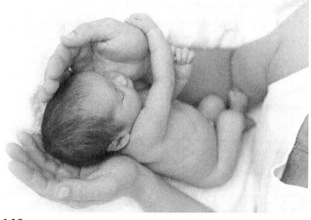

New moms are quick to judge themselves and need a kind, loving circle of support. Remember that there was a time, not too long ago, when sisters, mothers, aunts, grandmothers and other women in their community would surround new mothers.

There was a good reason for that. You may need to create that if you haven't stayed in the community you were raised in or if your family members aren't the network of support you need, for whatever reason

If a spouse or partner is consistently present, make sure you are both well-read on:

- Postpartum care instructions for Mom
- Newborn care
- Avoiding early breastfeeding challenges

Support

I F YOU DO not have 24-hour a day support in the home, I strongly suggest that you find a supportive and knowledgeable friend or family member that can stay with you for a few days. If there is no one around you that you feel comfortable with, find yourself a post-partum doula to help you through these first days. As with the labor doula, do not let cost inhibit you. Again, experienced support is ideal, but there are doulas-in-training that need hours to complete their certification and may work for free. The cost ranges from free (usually educated but lacking experience) followed by a steady upward climb based on years of service and diversity in experience. You may even find some independently wealthy, experienced postpartum doulas who have the freedom to volunteer. Some may barter for other services and many will accept payments over time. Make sure you are taken care of.

Limit visitors to those that will help you. No one who expects to be entertained or catered to is allowed. I mean it. The criteria for visitors are:

- people who will empty your dishwasher or do your dishes
- people who will take out your garbage
- people who will clean the toilet for you
- people who will bring you food

You are unlikely to want to let the world hold your new baby yet anyway so only invite people over who will take care you. You can repay the favor later—maybe you already have. Invite people who will meet your most basic needs, really well.

Heal

TAKE AT LEAST one full week of extremely limited mobility. Allow your milk supply to build and to allow your placental site and perineum to heal.

Uterus

IF YOU HAD a salad plate sized bleeding wound on the outside of your body you would take it easy, right? You can't see it, but it's there. Follow the guidelines given to you by your birth team and call them if you notice that bleeding increases. It may be within normal range, but an increase in bleeding or excessive clotting is your body's way of telling you that you are doing too much. Your uterus should remain firm (have your provider teach you how to find it and massage it if it is not contracted). Initially, it should be about the size, shape and feel of a grapefruit and is usually below the bellybutton.

Perineum

KEEP SWELLING AND discomfort down by alternating between icing your bottom and taking a warm/shallow Epsom salt sitz bath a couple times a day for the first couple days.

You can also use witch hazel pads or spray a little witch hazel on a sanitary pad and keep them in the freezer; it feels good and promotes healing. Some women also use oral Arnica to help treat bruising/tenderness that can occur.

Cesarean incision

YOU HAVE ALL the same intra-uterine healing to do as a non-surgical patient, and an additional healing site from the alternate exit. Follow post-operative instructions. Your recovery time is likely to be in the 6-8-week range. Many healthy women who happen to end up with a cesarean birth feel pretty good, pretty soon. If this is true for you, that is wonderful, but it doesn't mean that you can start training for the marathon just yet. Internally, your body needs to take the time to heal well. Spend your time focused on adoring your baby, he/she will only be a newborn for a short time and you have a medical mandate to really experience a huge percentage of that time. Take it!

Breastfeeding Tips for the First Days

AVOID MANY EARLY nursing challenges by nursing often. After the baby is born—if unmedicated or minimally exposed—you should have a few hours with a wide-eyed, curious, alert baby. Some are vocal; some are quiet. Insist on having some privacy during this time to get to know one another.

Experiment with nursing during this time, if you feel unsure about anything ask for help from your doula, nurse, midwife, or a lactation specialist. Soon, baby will get sleepy, and you will too. Following delivery, you get one freebie sleep. Just this once you can sleep until the baby wakes you. Take advantage of this. After this one freebie and until baby has recovered his/her birth weight, you must nurse every 2-3 hours around the clock. If you put this on project status it will get there faster, usually within a week.

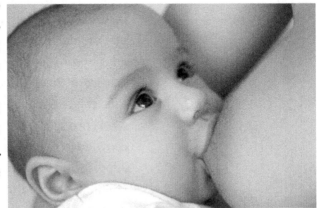

I know that it can be really hard. I know that you just want one more hour and that the baby may not be easily awakened, but the challenges of this time are not equal—not even close—to the emotional, physical and mental challenges you would face after your first postpartum visit if your care provider is worried about your milk production or your baby's growth. That, my friend, is stress. Avoid this issue if you can. Once the birth weight has been reached, you will continue to nurse frequently throughout the day, but can let your baby wake you at night, gently working toward nursing more during the day and less at night. Newborns should not sleep through the night. They need to eat, they need to grow; they need to triple their birth weight in the first year. They need to eat a lot.

Breastfeeding Basics

HOPEFULLY, YOUR BABY will be born with the strength and endurance to nurse, a good latch, and you will have no challenges, but it is healthier to expect a few bumps in the road and be prepared. It's rare to have issues that are insurmountable, but it often requires early conviction to reach the effortless comfort you may see in moth-

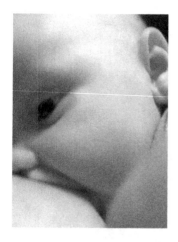

ers nursing at parks and shopping malls. Like every other subject we've discussed, understand that breastfeeding is not a guarantee for every woman or every child. There are medical, physical, emotional and developmental reasons that could prevent a woman from being able to breastfeed, rare though they might be. But again, I want you to be empowered and know the strength and beauty that your body possesses and is capable of giving to your child. I want families to make this important decision with information, not out of fear, unfair sexual/social beliefs, the cultural norms of family or friends, or total lack of information. Your child deserves for you to investigate both sides and make an informed decision. In fact, you deserve to know that from the beginning, from the first decisions that you make on your child's behalf, that you did your absolute best.

Throughout history, and to this day, formula companies acknowledge that their product is second best to breastfeeding. Consider the idea of *any* other product being marketed in this way. The idea of a healthy woman, with no breastfeeding complications, choosing to formula feed her baby is like ignoring a wild, abundant, organic garden in your backyard and buying your produce from a factory farm. Nursing your baby has incredible benefits. Here is the short list from La Leche League International, with additional editorial notes in italics, by me!

The 10 Easy Reasons to Breastfeed

1. Baby's whole body and brain benefit immensely.

    Breast milk is made specifically for your baby, with his or her specific nutritional needs realized by your body. It is pretty magical if you really think about it, your body knows what her body needs.

2. Release for mother hormonally causing calmer feelings.

    Prolactin, the hormone that allows you to sit and nurse your baby while all hell breaks loose around you, dishes, laundry, phones ringing, solicitors at your door. It's mother natures' way of telling you what is most important. It also helps you to relax and rest with your baby during the early weeks/months when you need to, to get enough sleep within a 24-hour period, cuz those 8 hours aren't happening in a row, during the night. Babies need to eat at night for healthy growth and development.

3. Easier digestion for baby than formula.

Breast milk is a live fluid and is therefore easily digested. It is also the perfect nutrition for your baby, so there is not a lot of "waste". BO-NUS! I would bet my life that if companies had to list GMO on the label, most, if not all, formula (as well as the "follow up food") labels would be wallpapered with warnings. It baby's first processed food.

4. Available fresh instantly for hungry baby.

No sterilizing bottles and nipples, no racks on your kitchen counter to dry all the sterilized equipment, no midnight bottle preps, no warming it to the right temp (your baby will very likely have a specific preference), no machines on your night table to keep it heated, no running out to convenience stores in the night, sometimes being forced to buy another brand that baby won't eat, no running out of prepared bottles on daytrips or at day care, or on the freeway in a traffic jam. Breast milk is always available, properly mixed and heated, and stored in a very accessible, beautiful container.

5. Soothing for a crying baby.

While it is important to build other comfort measures into your routine so Mom isn't the only one who can soothe a crying baby, and so that even Mom has other tools in her belt in case nursing isn't convenient, the reality is that nursing is soothing and will calm and quiet a fussy baby, even if she isn't crying out of hunger. Of course, it's ideal to make sure that she isn't crying because of another physical need, like burping, changing a diaper etc. before going straight to the breast every time. It is comforting to be at the breast, to be held. It is comforting to be fed. The action and stimulation of nursing can be soothing, and offers baby something else to focus on aside from whatever it was that was causing him to cry.

6. Treasure of a lifetime bond with your child.

Of course, you can have a lovely lifetime bond without breastfeeding. Time spent holding and singing to your baby are bonding activities. Breastfeeding offers some additional physiologic benefits. You have no choice but to give your baby your full attention at feeding time, there is no option to prop the boob and go do laundry. Additionally, the skin to skin contact increases your levels of Oxytocin (love hormone) as well as other hormones that can help you feel centered and calm.

7. Free (cheaper than formula by a long shot)!

So, this information is not easy to track down. If you chose the CHEAPEST formula to feed your baby and picked up bottles at goodwill *or used hand me downs, it's not that expensive, but still in $1000-$2000/ yr range. If you choose the most expensive brands and buy the newest trendy bottle that is BPA free, etc. you are looking at more in the $3000-$4000/yr range. I can think of so many other things to spend that money on, especially since your body makes its competition so effortlessly. I always encourage my clients to breastfeed for the minimum recommended by WHO (World Health Organization) 9 months to a year, and then use the leverage of how much money you've saved the family to go buy yourself a reward of some kind. My favorite idea is a shopping spree for all new, beautiful, sexy underwear. It's a classic win-win. Especially when you consider the next bullet point!*

8. Effortless pregnancy weight loss.

Assuming that you are eating a healthy, well balanced diet to build a supply of breast milk that is the best you can provide for your baby, any excess pregnancy weight gain will fall away, and you will soon realize that the fat that was once on your hips, appears to be chunky little rolls on his legs and making knuckle dimples on her hands!

9. Enhanced poop smells better than formula-fed babies (until solids start!).

Breast milk is so perfect that there is very little waste, and what waste there is, (if you are well nourished) doesn't consist of toxic chemicals and other unnatural ingredients that are difficult to digest. Formula poop stinks to high heaven. There is a lot of waste. Over the years it has been my experience that there is even a difference in the way the actual baby smells. There often is a metallic scent, sometimes subtle, sometimes distinct, to a baby whose diet is solely formula, while breastfed babies often have a naturally sweet, "new baby" smell until solid foods are introduced.

10. Decreased risk of SIDS than formula-fed babies.

There isn't any real proof that the formula is causing SIDS, there may be a number of lifestyle factors in play, but we shouldn't take a risk like this unless there are no other options. There are advocates trying to make it necessary to have a prescription for formula because of the risks it introduces and the health costs that are preventable with breastfeeding. Even if you have no choice but to supplement with formula, there are still incredible benefits in part time breastfeeding. For the first weeks and months healthy breast milk can prevent so many possible complications and has so many other benefits, I strongly encourage you to give it a chance and a solid effort. Did I mention that it's free?

The following address will take you to the La Leche League International's website for more information.

http://www.llli.org/nb/nbsepoct06p204.html

For those who may not have heard about La Leche League, or may have only heard about them in passing, I would like to take a moment to introduce them the way I do for my students in the classroom. La Leche League International is a highly acclaimed grassroots organization of (mostly) women. The root of the organization is to make sure women know everything that the founders wished they had known when they were beginning to breastfeed their own children. There was then, and still is a lot of misinformation, at times a total lack of information, false assumptions, fear mongering, sexual/social misunderstandings, and a new issue that this generation of new mothers face a ridiculous overabundance of data that makes it impossible to figure out what to expect, what to prepare for, what to do, what you need, what to buy, what to avoid, who to call for help or support, who to call for education etc. I hope to narrow it down for you.

So, your baby is born and you are planning to breastfeed.

Make sure that the support people around you are trained to help, as you and your baby learn to breastfeed. While it is one of the most natural things in the world to do, it is still likely that there will be a few bumps in the road, which are usually easily surmountable when you have knowledgeable support.

There are a lot of birth advocates, teachers and new or expecting parents out there that are really "into" immediate breastfeeding, meaning baby exits the vagina and latches as soon as possible. I only have one caveat to this idea; the baby is a participant and may not be interested immediately. It is beneficial to stimulate the breast/nipple by having baby "at" the breast. This causes an increase in oxytocin (love hormone discussed in earlier chapters) and can help the uterus to tighten, helping the placenta to detach and decreasing your risk of blood loss.

When possible, when everyone is healthy, it is wonderful to bring baby up to the abdomen and encourage him or her to find the nipple and latch on. I have seen *many* babies, however, who are simply not quite there yet. They may have some gunk to work out of their pipes, they may be exhausted after labor, they may be wide awake, alert, engaged and may just want to look into your eyes for a while. In my opinion, baby gets a vote. Your baby may show you that she is ready to begin breastfeeding by showing you hunger signs. These can range from a subtle sort of tiny lip smacking, to turning the head and opening her mouth, to a gaping mouth in a frantic search of something to latch on to. You can encourage your baby by remaining skin to skin, keeping baby near or at the breast, touching and tickling his cheek, stroking your finger across his lips and inserting a pinky finger gently into his mouth to play and coax. It should be noted that babies who have been exposed to narcotic and anesthetic medications during labor, especially for a prolonged period of time, will likely have effects after the delivery that can make breastfeeding (and bonding in general) difficult until the effects of the drugs wear off.

Once your baby is showing an interest in latching on, the current popular philosophy is the baby-led latch, meaning that the baby knows how to latch on if she is positioned at the breast in a way that lines up properly. Your baby should not have to turn his head to latch on; he should be positioned belly to belly and lined up so that his nose is opposite your nipple. The new concept suggests that with good positioning, while you are supporting the hips and shoulders making baby feel secure, she can latch herself. I think this is a wonderful place to begin; give thousands of years of instinct an opportunity to works its magic. This can be done in most any breastfeeding position. I prefer cross cradle position for new moms, but it can be done in football hold, cradle hold, or side lying.

A good latch has specific characteristics.

1. It doesn't hurt; you should feel a tugging, but no pain. Some mild discomfort can be normal, but the sensitivity should lessen throughout the feeding. If over a period of days, it becomes increasingly uncomfortable to nurse, or if there are cracks/fissures in the nipple or if the nipple comes out

of baby's mouth squished or otherwise misshapen, seek support.

2. Your nipple should be as far back in the baby's mouth as possible. Feel the roof of your own mouth with your own tongue. The ridged area right behind the teeth is the hard palate, keep moving back until you reach the space where the palate gets smooth and there is a considerable sloping increase in space. That is where you want your nipple, not smashed against the hard palate, but cradled in the soft, spacious cavern of the soft palate. You may need to break the latch by inserting your finger and re-latching until he gets it right, but I strongly recommend being as stubborn as hell on this one. *Even* if he is really hungry. *Even* if she cries when you remove the breast. Be patient and calm while you are both learning this new skill together.

3. Your baby's tongue should be under the breast, pressing the breast tissue behind the areola against the soft palate. The baby isn't exactly "sucking" she is milking the breast by compressing the ducts behind the nipple against the soft palate to eject the milk. Her tongue rolls from the tip, towards the back pressing the milk out. We can see the jaw gliding as she does this.

4. The lips should be flared out, not pursed tight around the nipple, they should be covering most of the areola, the darkened skin surrounding the nipple, (if not all of it) depending on the size.

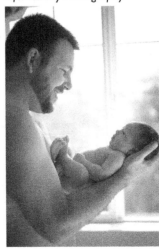

Life Actually Photography

5. For the first few days your baby is getting colostrum. The magical, concentrated, golden, protein rich, passive immunity infused, glorious substance that has so many benefits to your baby. The baby will have to work for it. There is not an unlimited supply and she will only consume a few tablespoons in the first days of life. Because it is thicker and she is learning to nurse, the suck to swallow ratio is around 7-10 sucks : 1 gulp/swallow

6. Once the milk comes in (usually by the 3rd or 4th day postpartum, but sometimes a little longer following a surgical birth or a longer labor) you should be hearing the gulping

and swallowing at a rate of 2-3 sucks : 1 gulp/swallow. Sometimes even 1 suck : 1 swallow, especially at "let-down" when the milk rushes at beginning of a feeding.

Now, as you can well imagine, it is not easy to know if all of the above factors are being done correctly, simultaneously. Also, just getting the baby positioned well at the breast can take more than two hands at first, so I am a big believer in both parents (when possible) being educated about breastfeeding. A nursing mom can't see underneath her own nipple. A nursing mom can't always see the baby's lower lip or the areola under the baby's mouth. A nursing mom can't always support the baby's hips and shoulders AND the weight of the breast for good positioning. It takes some teamwork for the first week or two, until the baby figures it out and there is muscle memory. If there isn't an available partner in the home 24-7, you might consider having a helper stay with you the first few days. A mother, sister, cousin or friend can be perfect if they are supportive of breastfeeding and aren't going to push a bottle every time the baby cries or moves or squeals or looks hungry.

Burping

If your baby is showing signs that he needs to be burped—grimacing, squirming, crying after a feeding, etc.—there are many techniques that can be used and your baby will probably have one particular position that works best. A firm stoke/pat guiding the gas bubble up and out with some pressure against the baby's abdomen (shoulder, forearm, hand, depending on what position you choose, will bring up those uncomfortable gas bubbles and relieve baby's pain. This, among other tasks, is a perfect opportunity for dads/moms/partners to acquire some one-on-one time together with the baby that is separate from breastfeeding. Use burping as an opportunity to gain an audience with your baby! In class, when I talk about this, I think it sounds somewhat cliché, and like somewhat of a boobie prize, pardon the pun, but my honey took this opportunity every chance he got. He gained a lot of confidence as a parent in being able to take care of seemingly simple things. Gas can be more of a challenge than you might think.

Common Concerns for Partners

Having a partner available 24/7, who is understanding, helpful and involved is something that I wish for EVERY new mama. I rarely meet with new parents without some mention of a newly realized and profound respect for single mothers. Having a calm supportive presence is so important. Do not underestimate the value of just being there. Nursing, even when uneventful is challenging at first, she is learning a new skill, and so is baby. Like labor, not knowing what "normal" is, can be hard by itself. Partners are in a unique position to support and be involved in successful breastfeeding. There are a few common concerns that I hear in my classroom and from new parents at our meetings following births that I'd like to address.

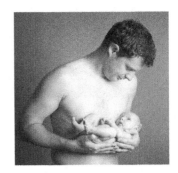

You may be worried about the baby interrupting the intimacy between you and your honey. In my experience and opinion, letting breastfeeding interrupt intimacy is a choice, as with most challenges that come up in a relationship. If you become educated about nursing, support each other, help with nursing challenges, protect and speak out in defense/support of her, compliment each other's strength and conviction, create your own unique and special bond with the baby without competing with the breast, I strongly believe that your intimacy can grow and deepen through breastfeeding.

I know that you may feel concerned about breastfeeding changing how you, or she, will feel about her breasts as related to sex or how breastfeeding will affect your sex life in general. Ok, so at first, while they are tender and she is getting used to this new nurturing role her breasts are playing, it may be true for a while. There will come a point, once the baby is nursing well, once her hormones have had a chance to balance, once she can have a bit of time between the nurturing act of breastfeeding and the expression of love and sexuality, she will be able to balance the two roles and know that her body is more than capable of both. Hopefully you will both experience a deepening respect and appreciation for the amazing breasts. They are beautiful, and provide nourishment.

Like intimacy, creating time, space and energy for sexuality becomes a choice. Everything is less spontaneous when you have children. If you accept each other in this period of growth and change, it can become part of your evolution as a couple. Additionally, I firmly believe that partners who are supportive, allowing the breastfeeding mother to be both a nurturing mother, and a loving partner to her fullest potential, not allowing the nurturing mother in her to feel pitted against the loving partner in her, are more likely to inspire a growing, healthy intimacy in your love relationship.

I know that you may be worried about the baby sleeping with you and never leaving. Co-sleeping as a lifestyle is a choice that must be made by the whole family. Co-sleeping in the beginning, in my opinion, is purely a survival tactic. In the early days and weeks, the baby has to nurse *a lot*. She has to regain her birth weight and be making progress towards doubling that weight in the first few months. You can put the baby in a room down the hall with a state of the art monitoring system, but you will lose more sleep, or at least Mom will, probably both. The earliest hunger signs are usually silent, little smacking lips or a slight rousing, but will wake a nursing mom if she is nearby. Sometimes she will wake up *before* the baby moves a muscle when they are close to one another. This means no screaming baby waking up the entire household, it also means that the baby hasn't necessarily even awakened fully and can be quickly and quietly nursed back to sleep. It definitely means that the baby hasn't been whipped into an adrenaline frenzy trying to get your attention and won't require an hour to calm down, nurse and get sleepy again. You don't necessarily have to have baby in bed with you. Co-sleepers are equally effective, even a cradle or portable crib next to the bed in the first few weeks/months can serve the same purpose. Just don't be shocked if baby goes to sleep in the co-sleeper and is in your bed in the morning. Getting out of bed to lay a sleeping baby down may just be too much of a risk to a very tired Mommy. Keep the lines of communication open and make sure you are making these decisions as a family. There are many ways to compromise and meet everyone's needs.

I know that you may actually want to give the baby a bottle. It's somewhat hard wired at this point to want to participate in this way. There will likely come a time when that will be an option for you. In the beginning, if breastfeeding is the objective, it is best to not complicate the feeding process for mom and baby. Offering the occasional bottle can lead to supply issues for Mom, and I have no doubt in my mind that it does have a distinct probability of confusing the baby. Sucking from a bottle (whether it's formula or breast milk) is not the same as expressing milk from the breast. For personal wishes to give baby a bottle please wait until the baby is a pro at breastfeeding, usually at least six weeks. There are many other ways to be involved in the care of your baby. Just being present during feedings will, over time, allow the baby to associate you with the good feelings of being at the breast. You can also help to support the baby, provide a warm, relaxing environment, stroke the baby's head or hold his hand, sing to him, be there hold him immediately after the feeding. You can allow Mom, once she has experience and confidence, one on one time with the baby during feedings and be creative building you own unique bonding time with the baby with your own one on one time. Again, there is no one *right* way to do this. Allow her to follow her instincts and you follow yours, be open with each other and work together to make sure everyone's needs are being met.

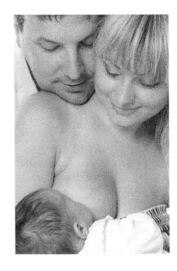

I know that you have much to offer as a companion through any breastfeeding distress. New mommies are sometimes…just a mess. The first days are somewhat of a roller coaster. She'll be exhausted from the birth. She may be exhausted from waking to nurse the baby around the clock. Her hormones may be fluctuating. Her body is changing and healing. She is adapting to the new overwhelming role of mother. When you add all of these together and then multiply that by our tendency to hold ourselves under a magnifying glass and compare ourselves to the "superwoman" our society idealizes, you can imagine that there may be a few emotional ups and downs. She will be grateful for you calm presence, your confidence in her, your confidence in her body, your being present as much as possible, your offering to help, your cool headed, methodical, if this, then that, then this again, problem solving attitude. She will value your patience and kindness.

As her partner, if you feel overwhelmed or if you think that she is overwhelmed, don't be afraid to seek help. You are our first, and sometimes only, eyes on her wellbeing in regard to the postpartum blues/depression continuum. If she doesn't seem like herself, if you feel worried, reach out to your birth team, they are still there for

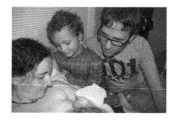

you. Even when there are no major concerns, it's normal to not always feel like you are qualified for this position, for both of you.

Again, if no one is able to fill this 24-7 support role for you, you can find a postpartum doula.

The following is an excerpt from an article about Postpartum Doula's.

What type of services does a Postpartum Doula provide?

The postpartum doula offers many services to her clients, but her main goals are to help "mother the mother," and nurture the entire family as they transition into life with a newborn. This would include doing things to help mom and dad feel more confident in their roles, sharing education on family adjustment and tending to the unique needs of a new mother.

A postpartum doula works with each family individually to find out their particular needs. Some of the duties that a postpartum doula will perform include:

- Breastfeeding support
- Help with the emotional and physical recovery after birth
- Light housekeeping so that mom does not feel so overwhelmed
- Running errands
- Assistance with newborn care such as diapering, bathing, feeding and comforting
- Light meal preparation
- Baby soothing techniques
- Sibling care
- Referrals to local resources such as parenting classes, pediatricians, lactation support and support groups

Most postpartum doulas provide service for a family anywhere from a few days up to a few weeks after bringing home a new baby. Families may have the doula work one to three days a week or as many as five days a week. Postpartum doulas often offer nighttime service to help the family transition more smoothly into the challenges of nighttime parenting. Each doula offers different services, so it's important that each family decide what their needs are and find a doula who can meet those needs.

Common pitfalls in early breastfeeding:

Nipple Shield: These damn things. I take that back. These things that have a VERY specific function, and are sent home with women constantly and (largely) needlessly. A couple reasonable uses for nipple shields are

1. There was an initial shallow latch that caused some nipple damage and the nipple needs a chance to heal before reintroducing nursing skin to skin.

2. Baby is having difficulty latching onto a flat or inverted nipple and the shield is meant to draw the nipple out while simultaneously stimulating the sucking reflex in the soft palate.

Like every intervention, it has a place. But they are handed out like candy (primarily in hospitals) and there is inadequate follow up. This tool is meant to be a very temporary band-aid for a very specific issue. Once the initial challenge is resolved, the baby still must learn how to latch onto the natural breast for successful, longer term nursing. The worst part about this tool is that it becomes a security blanket. If the baby becomes accustomed to the shield, he/she may become frustrated when trying to latch on without it. Mom's become frustrated, and sometimes even report feeling "rejected" by the baby.

Try to think of it more like teaching a child a new skill. New skills can be frustrating, if you spoonfed your baby because he was becoming frustrated trying to use the spoon himself, you are not demonstrating your confidence in his ability to do the new thing. If your daughter calls Spaghetti, Pascetti, and you never correct her, you aren't challenging her to learn and grow. New skills can be hard, and whether you nurse without a shield from the start, or have to take a slight step backward and begin again with your baby once the initial challenge has passed, you still have to go through the challenge of teaching your baby how to latch deeply, for everyone's best interest. If you are having a hard time, please contact La Leche League, or find a local lactation consultant who can guide you and support you as you learn to latch your baby.

Formula in the house: I know that new moms and dads are often on a billion mailing lists and that companies send out samples of products. If you have a sample of formula in the house, but intend to breastfeed, I am begging you, get rid of it. It is available at the store if you have an urgent need. It's the same concept as freezing your credit cards in a block of ice in the freezer; waiting for it to thaw gives you a chance to think about the purchase, it forces you to consider the consequences of an impulse decision. We all have moments of weakness, in the middle of the night, when we feel isolated and worried, when the baby is crying and we can't seem to console him or get him to nurse. I would much rather you wake someone up to ask for support than give the baby a bottle in a moment of weakness. Even if there is no one available in the night, just get through *that* night and seek skilled help in the morning.

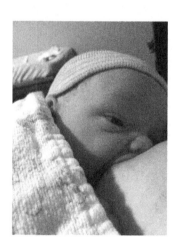

I know this is going to seem like a conspiracy theory, but why do you suppose formula companies send out samples instead of mailing out advertisements?

> A.   There isn't much to say about the product except that next to breastfeeding, it's the second best for baby. Umm, it's the only option next to breastfeeding, so that doesn't say much.
>
> B.   They know that the rate of return is worth the cost.

They are not assuming that you are going to taste it. It is not a gift. It is a trap. They know that once you give the baby formula, the challenges of breastfeeding increase. It's like the single ten-cent cigarettes they used to sell at the gas station. It's not that the substance itself is addictive in this case, it just becomes easier and easier to just satisfy the baby without a lot of effort, and it seems easy at first. Newborns don't require that much formula and it's like a novelty at first. Family members may even be encouraging it so that they can have a chance to feed the baby too. It will quickly have an effect on your milk production and then it will require more effort to rebuild your supply. It can be done, but the formula companies bet a lot of money on women giving up for good reason; many will. If you feel strongly about breastfeeding your baby, it will require some conviction, and not having any formula around makes it a lot easier.

Latching: Remember that in the first few days of life, the baby is getting colostrum and that is all she needs. Put it on project status in the first days to learn the right latch, so that once the milk is in you are not fighting this battle. If once the milk is in, you are still struggling with getting the baby latched on well, seek help. A poor latch that goes uncorrected can cause a litany of other issues in the first weeks. Occasionally there may be an anatomical reason for a poor latch, but most of time it is caused by the lack of understanding what it should look like ahead of time, and a lack of will to make sure baby latches correctly every time. Make sure you know what a good latch looks like.

Engorgement: Becoming engorged creates challenges for you and for your baby. If you are nursing around the clock, every two to three hours in these first days, until baby regains her birth weight, you may prevent engorgement from happening at all, or lessen the inflammation by keeping the breast tissue relieved from the pressure of milk in the ducts. Engorgement can lead to other problems, it can make it difficult for the baby to latch on and get enough breast in her mouth to be able to nurse effectively, it can lead to plugged ducts and eventually to an infection. Prevention is your best bet. Nurse often with a deep latch. It may some take work and it may take some support, but the challenges you can prevent are worth a little interrupted sleep for the first few nights.

Lack of information: Just like in childbirth, preparation and knowledge can help you to prevent challenges so you never have to deal with it in the first place. Not knowing what is normal makes it impossible to know what is abnormal. For example, while you are learning to nurse, there are specific positions and techniques that may work better for women with larger or smaller breast size and different nipple characteristics. I know there are many books on the market about breastfeeding, and I'm sure many of them offer some good information. Personally and professionally, I always recommend *The Womanly Art of Breastfeeding* by La Leche League because I trust the source and I know that they are continuously researching and revising the material as new information is realized. Additionally, they offer a series of *free* classes and offer support for women and their families, without judgment, whether you are planning to nurse for a month or for years, whether you are nursing part time or full time, whether you are working or stay at home. It is an invaluable resource. Many women don't realize that there is free support through the La Leche League; it is a huge international organization that probably has a group in your area. If there isn't one, you can get support over the phone and perhaps once your own challenges have been resolved, you can begin a group to help support other women in your community!

If any challenges that come up are not being resolved by using the knowledge you gained from this class, if it is not resolved by the DIY suggestions in the *Womanly Art of Breastfeeding*, and it is not being resolved by a consultation with a La Leche League Leader, either over the phone or in person, and it is not being resolved by a postpartum doula (if you have one), who ideally has some breastfeeding support training, then I recommend that you seek *kind* support from a trained lactation support/specialist/consultant. It costs a little money up front, but won't cost nearly as much a formula will over time. I would encourage you to interview over the phone and get a good idea about the philosophy of the person on the other end. Do you feel respected and supported? Do you feel like this person is really convicted to helping you find a solution?

Remember that you are not alone, by the time you are in this position you will have a circle of support around you, which will help guide you to the right path. If you have done your job well up to this point and surrounded yourself with supportive, patient, kind, people and medical professionals, you have built a diverse circle of wisdom. It is not necessary for you to prepare for step Z, because steps A-Y have already built a community that will be there to support you and your family. In the rare instance, if after all that you are unable to breastfeed, or breastfeed solely, then what I hope for you is that you will be able to be kind and compassionate to yourself, it is one of the most important lessons you can teach your child. Be consoled by the fact that you did everything in your power and you can feel released from the stress and the discomfort and the social pressures and the feelings of inadequacy and accept yourself and your child, with all your perfections and imperfections. Accept the reality of your situation; redirect your attention to other ways to build a beautiful bond with your child. Breastfeeding alone will not define your relationship. You and your child will have a million opportunities to do that together.

Normal Weight Gain:
- back to birthweight by day 7
- 7-10 ounces per week the first 4 months
- double birth weight by 4 months: a gain of 7.5 pounds-10.75 pounds
- 3.5-5 ounces per week month 4 to month 12
- triple birth weight by one year: a total gain of 15 pounds-21.5 pounds

  Source: 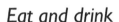http://www.thenewbornbaby.com/. Visit their site for more information!

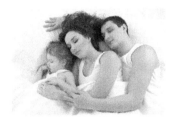

Eat and drink

YOUR BODY NEEDS to stay well hydrated and nourished to heal and create a milk supply for your baby. Make sure you have water (and snacks) at hand, especially when you sit down to nurse. You will be there for at least 20-30 minutes and will probably become progressively dehydrated/thirsty and hungry throughout the feeding. If you haven't had a baby shower yet, I love the idea of having everyone bring a freezable dinner and/or healthy snacks in addition to or instead of a gift. After all, baby clothes and toys are so easily available online and are also really fun to shop for. Ask for food, or housekeeping, making your time at home more focused on adoring this new little girl or boy. Even if you have a spouse at home, you should both spend your time bonding, not cooking and cleaning.

Bond

BONDING IS TIME spent connecting with intention. Breastfeeding women sometimes seem to have an advantage here. You get a captive audience during feedings, and very often, nursing is a source of comfort for both baby and mom. It isn't the only way to gain a captive audience, and it is not the only way to create a comforting relationship. Create other rituals. It doesn't all have to be about food. There is a lot of comfort in things that are routine. If you spend enough time with your baby, getting to know the little noises and faces and movements and cries, you begin to understand her. Talk to your baby. Tell her about your day, share family stories; tell him about your life, babies are great listeners. Listen to music or sing to your baby. You can sing anything you like, it doesn't have to be Brahms's Lullaby or Row Row Row your Boat. The songs you sing will become memories over time and your child(ren) will know you better. My Dad sang "Goodnight Irene," "Daisy Bell" (the bicycle built for two song), and one other crazy song called "The M.T.A." Unconventional lullaby, but I love this song; it's a special memory and will be there long after my Dad can't sing it for me anymore. My Mom sang: "Do-Re-Mi" and "My Favorite Things" from Sound of Music and a song from Sesame Street, "Sing a Song." I love that song, it makes me smile, inside and out.

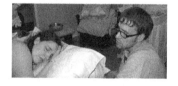

More bonding activities: make faces at him, he may copy you; it's a form of communication. Rock, bounce, sway, dance, massage, walk, play with toys, read books. Even watching TV with your baby has bonding opportunities. Spend time; it is such a gift. It feels slow when you are in it, but you won't believe how quickly you become one of "those people" who tell other new parents on the street how fast the time passes and to cherish every moment. It's truly bewildering. You can't help but miss the newborn, the infant, the baby, the toddler, the child, that he or she has already been, and never will be again, even as you delight and worry about the stage they are in, and look forward to all that is to come.

Use your time well.

Sleep

YOU DON'T HAVE to sign up for a lifetime of co-sleeping; there are as many opportunities to wean the baby out of your bedroom as there are days. In these early days, however, it falls into the category of survival. Keeping baby very near to you (in your bed, in a co-sleeper, or in a bassinet next to your bed) will allow you to meet his needs in the night without having to really fully awaken, climbing out of bed, walking down the hall, rocking and nursing and changing and nursing and rocking again, then walking back to bed. You can simply bring baby into your bed and nurse (keeping a stash of diapers and other tools bedside), change diaper (if necessary) and nurse back to sleep. If you can catch the early hunger signs, which would require you to be very close by, baby doesn't get to the point of having to cry to get your attention. Once she is crying, she will likely be wide awake and it will take longer to get her calmed down and back to sleep.

Sleep is also critical for the parents providing nighttime care. Newborn babies normally sleep between 16 and 20 hours a day, but it is intermittent sleep: 45 minutes here, 2 hours there, etc. If you are careful to sleep at least 8-10 hours in every 24-hour daily cycle, you should be able to function pretty well. Get as much sleep as you can at night, keeping baby near you so you can meet his needs efficiently, then nap a few times during the day with your baby. As previously discussed, newborns should not be sleeping through the night, anyway.

Even after they get back up to their birth weight and beyond, they need to eat at night to grow at a healthy rate. As babies grow, I see a lot of families who very quickly cling to any sign of a perceived sleep schedule or routine. I also see a lot of families trying "sleep training" tools. I'm going to be straight with you, I don't believe in them. There are rare cases of severe sleep issues that may benefit from some sleep training, but most babies go through normal fluctuations and phases. Whatever you try, any kind of routine may work for a while, but babies change, a lot. Their needs change, they begin teething, they have colds, they grow and need to nurse more often, they sleep well for a while, and then cut another tooth and the whole routine is in the toilet. Be cautious about jumping on board the "she is sleeping through the night" plan... you'll jinx yourself in a hot second. Parenting is not for the fainthearted, there are many nights of fitful or intermittent sleep in your future, sleep challenges and other challenges that will stretch your very soul, but few elements of life offer us the opportunity for personal growth and the depth of relationship that parenting will.

My wishes for you

I WISH FOR you a beautiful birth experience that—no matter the environment and level of support—you can look back on warmly, that will give you a sense of accomplishment in making the healthiest possible choices for your child, for yourself, and for you family.

I wish for you conviction in your expectation of being treated with dignity, respect and sincere care. Expect kindness, and don't settle for less. That is your new barometer: treat me with kindness or simply don't treat me at all. Vote with your dollars or with your insurance company's dollars. There is no need for a conflict; there are almost always other options.

I wish for you a sense of confidence—born out of this experience—that will allow you to advocate for yourself, your children, your partner, your parents, your friends. There will probably be times when it may be awkward to challenge an authority figure—your children's teacher, a principal, a boss, a spiritual leader, a doctor, a dentist, etc.—for you or for the benefit of someone you love. I have personally had to challenge all of the above. You have to ask questions and wait for informed, thoughtful, thorough answers. Wait patiently. People, who are considered "experts" or are seen as authority figures (and enjoy the perception), may not appreciate your inquisition. Be as kind as you can, but don't back down until you have the information you need.

I wish for you and your family a simple, loving, compassionate, fun, fulfilling, rewarding, comfortable life together, filled with enough of everything you need. Not too much, just enough. Your relationships will be what will matter at the other end of this journey.

As I write this closing, I have a candle lit (as is my custom) for all these wishes.

The candle is for you and for your family.

Namaste

Resources

Suggested Continuing Education for Parents:

Red Cross. Become certified by the Red Cross in Infant and Child First Aid and CPR. It will give you peace of mind knowing that if something happens, you will know what to do.

The Baby Book by Dr. Robert Sears and Martha Sears R.N. No one should enter into parenthood without this incredible resource. Everyone says, "I wish babies came with an instruction manual." Well, they do, but it's not included in the original packaging. You have to purchase it separately, like batteries. Considering its size, you'll be quite happy to buy it separately. Don't be intimidated by its size. It is a big book, but the section dealing with preparing for a new baby and the immediate care of a new born baby is about 1/8ᵗʰ of the book. It is a totally manageable amount of reading. I love this resource because of the editorial format. There is no judgment, just information. It's written in a common sense, easy to understand language and is organized to keep it simple and approachable. Dr. Sears, has authored, or co-authored a number of other books that I have valued over the years, but this is the one to buy first.

La Leche League. The Womanly Art of Breastfeeding. La Leche League is the first, and usually the last stop that a breastfeeding woman needs to make for breastfeeding support. Find this book and keep it near you while nursing. You can answer so many questions for yourself. For anything you can't answer, you can find a local La Leche League group by looking for their schedules online and ask them in person at a meeting. If there isn't a local chapter near you, the leaders are available by phone for consultation as well, and most of the time, their support is free. If there is a meeting near you, it can be a wonderful place for you to meet other like-minded families and receive support for any challenges you may be facing. You may be surprised how quickly you move from being the supported, to being the supporter, and that can be incredibly rewarding. This is a perfect opportunity to take a challenge, overcome it with support, and then make it purposeful by being there for someone else in her moment of need.

Citations

I am grateful for the resources I have quoted, referred to and suggested. For your convenience, here is a concise list.

Kennell, John H. MD. Your quote about the doula role has had a profound effect on my profession.

Erdoes, Richard and Ortiz, Alfonso, editors. American Indian Myths and Legends. "Brule Sioux Sun Creation Myth." Pantheon Books. 1984.

Ribary, Erika. Erika has been a student, sitting in my own childbirth education classroom. She has been a protégé, as she studied to become an educator herself. She has been a colleague, teaching childbirth education and providing labor support. And finally, she has been a mentor and a teacher for me, showing me that I could break away from the traditional certification and create my own path. Now retired from the birthing community, I hope she will accept my sincere gratitude and wishes for her continued success in her current and future pursuits.

Sears, William, M.D. and Sears, Martha, RN. The Baby Book. Little, Brown and Company. 2013. The most important book for parents to have on their nightstand and/or coffee table. This work is brilliant, editorial, thorough, concise, supportive and kind. There are so many resources provided by this family of real care providers. I am so grateful to be able to refer them all.

Beattie, Melody. The Language of Letting Go. Hazelden. 2009. I was first introduced to this book when I was going through the certification process to become a chemical dependency counselor in the early 1990's. Her quote on page 23 has a lot of special meaning to me.

Yoga. I thank all the instructors, video's and resources that contributed to the culmination of the breathing technique that I recommend for women both preparing for labor and in labor as a means of coping with contractions, encouraging tranquility and simultaneously providing the oxygen that her body and her baby need throughout this process.

American Pregnancy Association, Effects of Epidural Anesthesia. http://americanpregnancy.org/labornbirth/epidural.html.   This article confirms what most care providers are reluctant to admit. The placenta is not a barrier and does not prevent drugs from crossing into the baby's bloodstream. The drugs put into Mom's body can have effects on the baby well after the machine is turned off and the baby is sent home. The article cited the following resources.

American Academy of Family Physicians, http://www.aafp.org.

Harms, Roger W., M.D., et al, Mayo Clinic Guide To A Healthy Pregnancy.

Cunningham, F. Gary, et al. William's Obstetrics. Twenty-Second Ed.